Silently Seizing

Silently Seizing:

Common, Unrecognized and Frequently Missed Seizures and Their Potentially Damaging Impact on Individuals With Autism Spectrum Disorders

An Essential Guide for Parents and Professionals

Caren Haines, RN

With Valuable Input From Nancy Minshew, MD

Special Chapter: A Psychiatrist's View

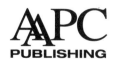

PUBLISHING
P.O. Box 23173
Shawnee Mission, Kansas 66283-0173
www.aapcpublishing.net

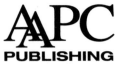

PUBLISHING
©2012 AAPC Publishing
P.O. Box 23173
Shawnee Mission, Kansas 66283-0173
www.aapcpublishing.net

Publisher's Cataloging-in-Publication

Haines, Caren.

Silently seizing : common, unrecognized and frequently missed seizures and their potentially damaging impact on individuals with autism spectrum disorders : an essential guide for parents and professionals / Caren Haines ; with valuable input from Nancy Minshew. -- Shawnee Mission, Kan. : AAPC Publishing, c2012.

p. ; cm.

ISBN: 978-1-937473-08-2 ; previous ISBN: 978061546702
LCCN: 2012944091
"Special chapter: a psychiatrist's view."
Includes bibliographical references.
Summary: A new way to look at some autistic behavior as the result of seizures rather than the autism itself. Includes up-to-date research and practical strategies.--Publisher.

1. Autism. 2. Epilepsy. 3. Nervous system--Diseases--Treatment. 4. Autism in children--Treatment. 5. Autism spectrum disorders--Treatment. 6. Anticonvulsants--Therapeutic use. I. Minshew, Nancy. II. Title: Seizures and their potentially damaging impact on individuals with autism spectrum disorders.

RC553.A88 H35 2012
616.85/882--dc23   1208

Disclaimer

This book is intended to aid those who love and care for a person with autism, to help them become essential, effective advocates and excellent observers of behavior. It is not a substitute for the guidance of medical professionals but an adjunct to the arsenal needed to help unravel the mystery known as autism.

Cover concept by Pamela J. Hunter
This book is designed in Myriad.
Printed in the United States of America.

CONTENTS

ACKNOWLEDGMENTS

I would like to give heartfelt thanks to all of those who supported and encouraged me on this project, beginning with my gentle and loving son Josh, who reminds me every single day to remain courageous in the face of any and all adverse circumstances. Josh, your incredible purity of spirit and your gentle, loving soul inspires me to leave no stone unturned in my quest to help you and serve your purpose in this life. I am forever yours.

Thank you to my wonderful husband, Chuck, and my beautiful daughter, Alyssa, for being simply the best of the best. To my loving and devoted friends, I need not name you; surely, you know who you are! To my exquisite and exceptional friends, Gail and Carol, you both know how much I adore you. We have traveled this dark and scary road together for so many years; I can't imagine my life without your love and support. You are one with my heart and soul.

I would also like to thank the fine physicians who assisted me on this project, Drs. Nancy Minshew, Darold Treffert, Fernando Miranda, Manuel Casanova and Holmes Morton. I am grateful for the insights you so generously shared. Your vast knowledge, gleaned through years of medical practice, and your commitment to share it with the readers of this book, is a gift beyond measure.

Dr. Minshew, your knowledge has forever changed our lives. You have given us hope for a brighter future for our children. You truly are an angel among us.

Dr. Morton, you are a wonderful country doctor who thoroughly understands the seizure-autism connection.

Dr. Treffert, thank you for your wisdom, caring and kindness. You are a treasure.

Dr. Linden and Dr. Miranda, thank you for adding valuable information that will help our readers.

Special thanks to psychiatrist Dr. Kanchun Mahon, who witnessed Josh's seizures in her office and emphatically and undeniably diagnosed him with temporal lobe epilepsy.

A special thanks goes to the physicians at Columbia Presbyterian Hospital in New York City. The team of esteemed physicians in the neuropsychiatry department headed by Dr. Agnes Whittaker continues to show our family great patience and understanding. Although they are skeptical about invisible seizures, they always try to keep an open mind, which led to successful treatment of these debilitating symptoms. For that I will be forever grateful.

A heartfelt thanks to the editorial magicians who worked tirelessly on this book, Anne Horton and Terri Daniel, to whom I am exceedingly grateful, and to Diane Goble for extraordinary research and Pamela Hunter for the concept of the beautiful cover.

A very special thanks to author Donna Williams, who gave us tremendous insight into the world of autism, which, despite so much research, we still struggle to understand.

Finally, a word to all the parents who find themselves in the same circumstance and struggle to find answers – leave no stone unturned in your quest to help your precious children. It is a labor of love. This book wouldn't be possible without the contributions of the beautiful families who allowed us to peek into their lives.

FOREWORD

The information in this book is based on work by a dedicated group of parents focused on helping others understand a complex and misunderstood dual diagnosis – autism and epilepsy. These parents realized their children with ASD (autism spectrum disorders) had undiagnosed seizures that manifested in abrupt onset of irritability, rage, twitching eyes, hallucinated smells, headaches and episodes of staring blankly into space. As a result of their extreme perseverance and desire to help their children, these parents were able to find a few physicians who were willing to guide them to the proper diagnosis and medications that led to remarkable overall improvements.

This book reflects the tremendous challenges and suffering that can result when medical issues in a misunderstood disorder fall at the intersection between two subspecialties, in this case neurology and psychiatry. This intersection can be an occasion where experts meet to solve unusual problems, or it can become a no man's land. It seems to be the latter.

Silently Seizing represents a first step on a path that needs to be explored. The information shared in these pages should be taken seriously by parents and professionals so that knowledge will be expanded for us all. It was assembled by the tireless efforts of Caren Haines and the families she interviewed, all of whom are on the front lines of autism and are determined to help their children become the best they can be.

The great difficulty is that those who are most familiar with the behavior of autism – psychologists, behavioral specialists, speech-language pathologists and child psychiatrists – often have little or no familiarity with the presentation of seizures other than those of a classic grand mal seizure. Further, there is a tendency to attribute all behavior that occurs in a person with autism to the impairment without attempt to dissect the origin. On the other hand, the neurologist who may be very familiar with epilepsy is likely to have little familiarity with the behavior of individuals with autism and intellectual disability. Also, there is an underestimation of the effect that many psychotropic medications have on the seizure threshold and an overvaluing of any given electroencephalogram (EEG), which is frequently of inferior quality and not utterly reliable when seizures are the subclinical variety; that is, a disorder that cannot be identified in a clinical setting. This leaves us with a huge gap between two diagnoses that are inextricably related to one another . . . seizures and autism.

The mode of detection is hotly debated, as many doctors see the EEG as the final word. Yet, what is *not* at issue is that epilepsy in those diagnosed with autism occurs at rates far above the general population, and the rate of abnormal EEGs is several times the rate of epilepsy, depending on the age of the children tested and the quality of the EEG. The current focus of EEG research in autism is on determining whether the abnormal electrical discharges, called *interictal spikes*, that can occur between seizures, are associated with cognitive and/or behavioral consequences.

You will be able to easily assimilate the information found here, and as a consequence, be better able to report accurately to your doctor what you are witnessing in your child. We hope the professional world will pay more attention to this perplexing problem and devote increased time and energy to helping these children lead more normal lives.

Nancy Minshew, MD

INTRODUCTION

A World Turned Upside Down

I felt motivated to write this book based upon my experience as a mother on the front lines of autism for more than 20 years. In my estimation, and with the agreement of some expert physicians, my son likely suffers from difficult-to-recognize partial seizures along with his autism diagnosis. On this journey, I have gathered information that might improve the outcome for the alarming number of children who are being diagnosed with autism every single day.[1] I hope this information finds its way into the hands of all parents facing an autism diagnosis in their child, especially those with a recent diagnosis, who can benefit the most from the help.

My son, Josh, was diagnosed with autism at the age of 2 years and 10 months, and all of his odd behaviors were deemed a part of this perplexing condition. Many of Josh's abnormal behaviors – screaming, pulling his hair out in clumps, staring spells and speaking gibberish – were misinterpreted as the "self-stimulatory" behavior typical of autism. Based on this diagnosis, my family was just supposed to grieve the loss of the normal child we would never have; accept it and move on.

What we know now, but did not know then, is that these behaviors can also be signs of partial epilepsy – a seizure disorder that can be difficult to recognize. Many people miss the more subtle signs seen in this condition and, therefore, miss the opportunity for early diagnosis and treatment, which is crucial to ensure the best possible outcome.

---

1   *A child with autism.* http://www.child-autism-parent-cafe.com/a-child-with-autism.html

My intention in writing this book was to let parents know that many of the troubling behaviors they're witnessing in their children are generally categorized by the medical community as symptomatic of autism, but they may also be caused by "stealth" absence or partial seizures that can be easily treated. An *absence seizure* can produce a blank stare, involuntary movements and chewing movements of the mouth, and may only last a few seconds. A *partial seizure* may begin with jerking of one area of the body, arm or leg, often while the patient is awake and aware. A more complex version, called *complex partial*, starts with a blank stare followed by chewing movements of the mouth. The person can mumble gibberish and seem to be in a trance. This kind of seizure can produce aggression.

Many of the behaviors the seizure generates subside with treatment. But untreated, these seizures can cause brain damage, which can lead to serious harmful effects such as self-injury and psychosis later in life. Therefore, the seizures must be recognized and treated early to preserve the function of the developing brain. However, if your child is older and has become self-injurious or psychotic, it's not too late for intervention. A protocol of medicine described in this book has worked for my son and other children so effectively that the episodes are almost extinguished. Some children are getting treated early and actually lose the diagnosis of autism altogether.[2]

It is my greatest wish that other parents of children with autism will find this book and be spared some of the suffering and confusion that we, and our precious children, have had to endure. I hope my experience will inspire parents to do their own research and educate themselves thoroughly about their children's diagnoses, rather than just accept what is told to them. It is important to dissect and analyze the child's behaviors so they can be accurately described

2   Shipman & Naltz (2008).

to the doctor and diagnosed as seizure-related. If an unrecognized seizure disorder is the underlying issue that is causing the constellation of symptoms we call "autistic," then treating it could produce a miracle of healing.

CHAPTER 1

JOSH'S STORY

When Josh was placed in my arms moments after he was born, I gazed into his beautiful blue eyes. I recall feeling that life does not get any better than this. I thanked my lucky stars for this perfect little blessing. Later, when the nurses shouted out "hypospadius!" as they assessed his every nook and cranny, the delivery room doctors and nurses reassured me that the condition, an abnormal opening of the penis, is "fixable."

Relieved, I returned to bathing in the bliss created by the arrival of my sweet angel. They brought him to me swaddled in a blue and yellow polka-dotted cotton blanket and tiny yellow cap. He was the sweetest sight imaginable, as he looked around wide-eyed at the marvel of new beginnings.

Josh's early childhood seemed normal. But between 18 months and 2 years, those few coveted words he had acquired – "Stop,""up,""ball" and "juice" – were uttered less and less frequently. It was as though a water faucet was being turned off in slow motion. Instead of flowing out of him, language appeared to be flowing away from him. I began to notice that for seconds to minutes at a time my beautiful toddler would stare off in a distant, hypnotic gaze. For the duration of the "spell," nothing I said could penetrate his gaze or divert his attention.

As a result of these changes, we had Josh tested by a series of medical professionals. First we went to an audiologist, wondering if Josh was losing his hearing. During the testing, Josh sat in a chair in a cold, sterile, sound-proofed room with an enormous pair of black headphones on his tiny head. As sounds beeped on one side and then the other, he clearly seemed annoyed by the noises. He could definitely hear. Once he exited the room, he smiled and giggled, as he often did, in response to all sorts of stimuli unseen to the rest of us. We wondered what he was thinking about. I longed to understand him.

Next, Josh was evaluated by a speech pathologist. Despite Josh's protests, she did a litany of tests without me in the room. When Josh emerged, he looked sleepy, and he was clutching his little blanket along with a new label ... "Speech delay of one year." It didn't sound terribly ominous, so it was a label we adjusted to, taking it on like a heavy new sweater we would dutifully wear. I felt I could deal with it.

But there were still so many things I wanted to know. Why didn't Josh respond when I called his name? Why did he like to lie so close to the wall, facing it for hours on end while laughing? Why did he take me by the hand to the pantry and throw my hand up to the cabinet to get me to open the door? Why didn't he wave bye-bye or want to play peek-a-boo? Why did he drop to the floor periodically and just scream? Why did he love to spin in a circle until dizziness hurled his tiny body to the floor? Why didn't he point to objects in an attempt to learn about his environment, like every other kid his age? Why didn't he sleep at night instead of jumping on his bed, endlessly giggling until the sun rose?

Could Josh's Behavior Be Caused by Seizures?

I was also very worried about Josh's continual staring spells, up to 50 or more in a day. Each episode lasted 5 to 30 seconds and, although they were brief, they were very intense. When Josh was 2 years and 8 months, I finally took him to see a neurologist. Dr. Ingrid Taff, a well-respected neurologist in Great Neck, New York, performed a standard test for epilepsy: an electroencephalogram, commonly called an EEG. This test measures and records the electrical activity of the brain through sensors (electrodes) attached to the outside of the skull and hooked up to a computer. The computer records the brain's electrical activity on the screen or on paper.

Josh definitely didn't like this, pulling the electrodes off as quickly as we tried to put them on. But we prevailed. The test was performed, and the results were normal. In retrospect, this makes sense, since he was not having one of his staring spells during the test. I since learned that an EEG only records what's happening in the brain at that moment.

Still, the doctor felt that the spells were compelling enough to warrant a trial of anticonvulsant drugs. She described a seizure as a temporary short-circuit of the brain, which can cause physiological and behavioral changes. She suspected a specific type of seizures in Josh, "absence seizures," which are caused by a misfiring of electrical impulses deep inside the brain's temporal lobe (see Chapter 4), the part of the brain where much of language development originates.

Dr. Taff believed that the EEG could have failed to pick up Josh's seizures. Thus, she encouraged us to treat the seizures even though Josh's EEG was read as normal. Once Josh was stable on a proper dose of an antiseizure drug, such as Carbamazepine (Tegretol), she thought he would begin to speak and learn.

The words "speak" and "learn" were like honey pouring over me. I drank them in desperately and prayed that the doctor was right about the diagnosis of seizures. Imagine, hoping and praying for such a thing! That is how devastating some of the alternatives felt. If Josh had something that could be treated with medications, we could move forward with a more normal life. That would be wonderful! I felt the burden slowly lifting as she spoke. I had renewed hope.

One Step Forward, Two Steps Back

Josh was prescribed Tegretol to control his silent seizures. Unfortunately, within 24 hours of taking his first dose, he developed a head-to-toe, welt-like rash, so we took him off the medication immediately. The next day, by coincidence, he had a long-awaited appointment with a neuropsychiatrist who was, we had been told, an expert on developmental disorders.

The doctor pointed out that Josh made very limited eye contact and failed to respond appropriately to any requests. During the exam, Josh moved about the room singing a few words from the songs he had memorized from his favorite Raffi tape, "Baby Beluga la-la-la." He really seemed to be tuning out the world that day. As we watched the scene unfolding before us, the doctor asked about Josh's difficulty attending to any one specific task. He told us that, typically, children Josh's age (he was 2 at the time) use sentences to communicate and understand even more language than they use.

Watching Josh with what I thought was a measure of objectivity, I surmised that he must be very tired, a bit cranky from the itchy rash and maybe feeling a tad stubborn. But the doctor had a different take on it. He told us simply and clearly: "Your son, Josh, has autism."

I will never, ever forget that day. I could barely see the doctor's impassive face through my tears. As they fell in torrents on my shirt, I looked over at my then-husband, who was looking equally pained. The diagnosis was searing in its honesty.

The doctor went on to say, "These children have a lifelong developmental delay and have great difficulty adjusting socially. Most children with autism have some degree of intellectual impairment, and only about 20 percent have average or above-average intelligence."

He felt Josh had varying degrees of cognitive ability, with memory being one of his strengths.

With regard to the staring spells, this doctor thought they were likely an integral part of Josh's autism rather than a separate or treatable entity. We took his advice, discarding the idea of treating Josh's "invisible" seizures. In hindsight, I believe this was a tragic mistake.

Many years later, as I began to put together the pieces of our puzzle, I realized that Josh had a seizure disorder all along. As it progressed, its manifestations went well beyond staring spells. His more severe seizures produced vicious rage, undirected horrific violence and self-mutilating behavior, including bites that have left his skin forever scarred. Knowing what I know now, I agonize over a wish that I could somehow go back in time and change the choices I made.

Questioning Authority

We trust that medical professionals have profound understanding of the many human afflictions, and we trust them with our lives. Yet, there are times when it's difficult to obtain a clear, definitive diagnosis. Despite much progress, many human conditions remain a mystery in terms of the cause and a viable treatment. Autism and partial seizures fall squarely into this category.

Parents and caretakers of children with autism need to arm themselves with as much knowledge as they can possibly glean from those who have studied this perplexing disorder in depth. In particular, it is important to work with a team of experts who understand and treat the complexities of this disorder.

Unfortunately, we often rely on inexact science to tell us what is wrong with our children without questioning that science. This can lead to the erroneous assumptions we make as to why a child lashes out, screams or becomes violent, but the truth is we don't always know. The reason we don't know is that most of these children cannot answer the basic question, "What's wrong?"

How many of us have the tools we need to dissect the behavior of our children with autism? When we are told by experts, "this is just the way they are," we believe it, because as parents and average people we don't have the tools to look further. So we grieve the loss and go on with our lives, accepting that our children bang their heads for no reason, walk on their toes, cling to a wall in fear, cover their ears and stare into space. We believe that this is a part of autism, a disorder for which no existing remedy can significantly alter the course.

But what we – and many doctors – may not recognize is that these behavioral traits are also common manifestations of seizures in children. And untreated, these seizures can predispose children to develop similar types of behavioral disturbances, such as self-injury, aggression and psychosis, which are seen in many cases of autism.

When I went to the medical community seeking answers to my questions about the possible relationship between Josh's condition and a seizure disorder, initially I was met with staunch resistance and closed doors. Josh had started slipping away into brief dreamy episodes too numerous to count, and by age 12, these episodes had the added characteristic of uncontrollable aggression. It was a kind of madness in which strange, acrid smells lingered in his perception and odd voices screamed at him from inside his head. He told me he heard potato chip crunch sounds, and he covered his ears often. However, no one in the medical community listened to my theory that many years of brief partial seizures had morphed into a pattern of complex partial seizures (see Chapter 4), possibly underlying and exacerbating my son's autism.

And thus began my quest to understand the seizure connection as it relates to the diagnosis of autism.

Why didn't the doctors want to believe that Josh could be suffering an underlying syndrome of silent seizures? Why were they so willing to discard Dr. Taff's earlier assessment of a seizure disorder? Was it simply the lack of clinical proof that was causing disregard for what seemed to be so obvious?

In our continuing search for answers, various epilepsy experts ordered EEGs, and all showed normal results. Other tests were discussed, and some were performed, but no conclusive results emerged.

We now know that results of many of the tests used to detect seizures can be completely normal, despite a true diagnosis of epilepsy. Many experts agree that the diagnosis of a partial seizure disorder has to be made "clinically;" that is, based upon a description of the person's symptoms and the patterns in which they occur. This is precisely how Dr. Taff had diagnosed Josh years earlier.

"Please Fix My Brain, Mom!"

Back in the world of autism, many professionals who consulted on our case labeled Josh's odd behaviors (facial grimacing, eye blinking and fluttering) as "stims," a short term for *self-stimulatory behavior*. His habit of staring blankly into space for brief intervals throughout the day was given the euphemistic term of "light gazing." Once, as he was observed staring off into space, his eyes transfixed for about 30 seconds. A behavioral therapist surmised that this was Josh's way of internally stimulating himself. S~~omeone suggested that this~~ *divert attention* staring behavior is purposeful and has s~~ome benefit to him. She did~~ *- educacac usage.* *- Staring spells* ot take into consideration the possibilit~~y that these stims and spells~~ uld be manifestations of seizures.

The doctors told me that when Josh reached puberty, his behaviors could "get much worse," but nobody ever detailed what that might look like, so I was not prepared for what was coming.

Since conventional tests still did not register any signs of seizure activity, Josh's doctor at the time suggested that he probably suffered from a "mood disorder with psychotic features."[3] As a result, he was treated with high doses of antipsychotic drugs, including Risperidone (Risperdal), which was supposed to help relieve his "mood disorder." There was also speculation that Josh was experiencing a major depression, so additional medications were prescribed.

But the drugs given to relieve these problems made his behaviors much worse. This alone should have been a clue that something else was contributing to Josh's out-of-control behavior. For example, most of the time, he was capable of being extremely happy, gregarious and loving. In contrast, a person with a primary psychotic disorder (such as schizophrenia) is significantly lacking in emotional connection with others and appears out of touch with reality.

Schizophrenia vs. Depression

Schizophrenia is a serious brain disorder in which people abnormally interpret reality; it is characterized by a combination of hallucinations and delusions, with disordered thinking and behavior.

Depression is considered a serious medical illness that affects how a person thinks, feels and behaves.

These disorders can co-exist with autism, but treating any one of them in isolation will not achieve a remission of symptoms. All of the co-morbid issues need to be treated individually.

---

3   M. Nishawala (personal communication March 21, 2007).

Josh has been on his bed watching TV. Suddenly, he calls out profanities as he rudely asks someone, a hallucinated entity, to leave him the f*** alone. I run, trying to negotiate the stairs two at a time, so I can try to keep him from hurting himself.

His body is shaking, his pupils enlarge, and his shrill screams fill the air. His eyes glaze over as if he is possessed by some demon. "My eyes aren't working; my eyes aren't working, Mom!" Josh screams. Then the staring. No movement for about 30 seconds, eyes widened, as he is transported to a far-away place. "My brain is broken!" he bellows as he repeatedly taps his head.

Then his fear turns a dark corner. He becomes enraged. He lunges at me, and in a second, his hands are suddenly around my neck. I try to extricate myself from his grip as his anger intensifies. In the seconds that follow, he throws a punch with such force that it hurls me backward onto the floor. I clutch my face in pain and disbelief. My blood is everywhere.

"The Ninjas have guns," he growls and then begins to kick into the air while making combat-type sounds.

After a few more excruciating moments, the Ninjas retreat. Josh is panting and seems to settle down. He looks at the devastating scene of smashed objects, blood and broken glass around us. He sees me holding my face, sobbing. He surveys the mess with profound confusion and sadness, and asks me, "What happened, Mom?" Just then, my precious son, now 18 years old, who was diagnosed with autism at the age of 2 years and 10 months, actually apologizes. "I'm so very sorry, Mom. Can you give me a hug?"

I am reluctant in that moment out of fear, and I sheepishly refuse. He begins to sob with his head in his hands. He pleads with me, "Please, fix my brain."

As Josh's adolescence raged on, I continued to bring up to anyone who would listen the idea that Josh might be having seizures. By this time, I was certain that his symptoms mirrored those of temporal lobe epilepsy (see Chapter 4). But sadly, I was starting to sound like a broken record, and was beginning to be treated by the professionals as if I had lost my sanity.

Affirmation at Last

After years of relentless research, I eventually found a community of doctors and researchers who believe as I do that silent seizures are likely exacerbating autism in Josh and in many other children. I have talked with parents of children with autism who shared their belief that their children also suffer from invisible seizures. As a result, I have come to realize that many parents of these children are dealing with similar situations.

I know that many more children like my son are out there "silently seizing" because the scientific world has not yet fully embraced this perplexing connection. As I resolved to find out as much as I could about the intersection of seizures and autism, I was fortunate to gain critical knowledge from the expertise and support of several top medical professionals in the field of autism.

One of the extraordinary doctors I have come to know is Fernando Miranda, MD, a respected neurologist who has held prominent positions at Johns Hopkins University and the University of Maryland. Dr. Miranda is the founder of The Bright Minds Institute,[4] a groundbreaking organization dedicated to helping children with neurologic and learning disorders. Dr. Miranda speculates that as many as half of the children diagnosed with autism may be suffering from undiagnosed, difficult-to-recognize seizure disorders, resulting in the behaviors and symptoms we have come to call "autistic." Indeed, Dr. Miranda and a small number of other specialists are seeing impressive results treating these seizures in young patients previously diagnosed with autism.

I, along with many families, walked blindfolded through this maze of autism and seizure until very recently. Now, as the parent of an older child, I feel compelled to share what I have learned and to provide other families with a guiding light on what can be a terrifying journey. I know and understand first-hand how devastating it is to be told that one's beautiful child has an incurable, lifelong, neurodegenerative condition called autism. But once the diagnosis has been made and the tears have lessened, I must tell you that there is tremendous hope.

In hindsight, I realize that I missed an opportunity to diagnose and treat Josh's invisible seizures early on. By inadvertently allowing his brain to continue to silently seize, we robbed it of its ability to function normally. The brain is a miraculous organ that tries to find new neural pathways to help compensate for injury.

Josh is an artistic savant, meaning that he has a special skill that surpasses the skills of others who are not savant. This form of expression has allowed him to share the many struggles he faces with those who view his artwork. I often wonder if this amazing artistic skill, which appeared out of the blue and without any formal training, is his brain's way of compensating for the injury.

---

4   http://www.brightmindsinstitute.com

If Josh had been treated as a baby for his underlying seizure disorder, I believe his outcome would have been different. We lost valuable time that can never be recovered, as Josh's brain is now irreparably damaged by years of uncontrolled, erratic electrical activity, and yet he continues to make significant strides.

Thankfully, my son and I are past the daily rages that once forced me to contemplate placing him outside the cocoon of a loving home. It took nearly 10 years of trial and error, but finally the team found the right combination of medicines for Josh.

When children who are silently seizing are treated early with anti-seizure medications, many begin to show amazing gains in expressive language and comprehension. Many begin to speak and learn as many of their troubling behaviors disappear or greatly improve. Even more important for some of these children, an absolute miracle is occurring: They are losing their diagnosis of autism.[5]

Fortunately, we now live in a time when greater attention is being paid to the baffling origins of autism. There is much that can now be done to help these children once their underlying issues are fully understood.

---

5   F. Miranda (personal communication, May 5, 2009).

CHAPTER 2

WHAT AUTISM IS ... AND IS NOT

Most of us are aware of the dramatic rise in the diagnosis of autism over the past 10 to 15 years. The Centers for Disease Control and Prevention (CDC) reported in 2010 that autism spectrum disorders now affect an average of 1 in 110 children in the United States.[6]

Is the incidence of autism actually increasing in our population or is it just being recognized and diagnosed more frequently than in the past? If the increase is real, then what is causing it? Is it the additive that was once put into our childhood vaccines, which has been deemed toxic and since removed? Could it be that toxic chemicals have found their way into our food and water? Is it a proliferation of genetic mutations, some of them not yet detectable by conventional testing methods?

Speculation abounds regarding these questions and has been the subject of heated debate. One particularly controversial theory suggests that autism may be created in vulnerable people through exposure to a mercury compound (Thimerosal) formerly used as a preservative in childhood vaccines. This supposed link between autism and vaccination was fueled by simple, but inconclusive observation.[7] First, many children developed symptoms of autism dur-

6 http://www.cdc.gov/ncbdd/autism/data.html
7 Reynolds & Dombeck (2006).

ing the same period of time that they received the MMR (measles, mumps and rubella) vaccines. Second, mercury is a known toxic compound that can result in neurological damage in children and adults that appears symptomatically similar to autism. Despite the compelling simplicity of the alleged connection between autism and Thimerosal, the available research suggests that there is no reliable relationship between them.

I believe there are many sides to the autism story that have not been fully explored. This chapter will explain in brief what is known to be true about the origins of autism – what it *is* and what it is *not*.

Why Is the Number of Autism Diagnoses Increasing?

The number of reported cases of autism increased dramatically in the 1990s and early 2000s. This increase is largely attributable to changes in diagnostic practices, referral patterns, availability of services, age at diagnosis and public awareness,[8,9] though unidentified environmental factors cannot be ruled out.

In addition, a much bigger blanket has been cast over behavioral patterns that can be diagnosed as "autism." Physicians rely on a manual known as the *Diagnostic and Statistical Manual of Mental Disorders, 4th Edition* (DSM-IV-TR)[10] for the criteria that spell out how a mental disorder can be classified. Autism made its first appearance in the DSM in 1980. Meanwhile, in 1990, the Individuals With Disabilities Education Act (IDEA)[11] was introduced, mandating that children with autism receive special education services in the public schools. This mandate resulted in a jump in the number of diagnoses labeled autism.

---

8   Frombonne (2009).
9   Wing & Potter (2002).
10 American Psychiatric Association (2000).
11 National Dissemination Center for Children With Disabilities (2011).

In "The Autism Epidemic: Fact or Artifact?," psychiatrist Wazana and colleagues Bresnahan and Kline, all of the Department of Epidemiology, Mailman School of Public Health at Columbia University, point out that the average age of a child diagnosed with autism has gradually gotten younger – from about 7 years in 1987 to 3 years in 1994 – thus, creating a large jump in the number of overall cases.[12]

With the rules of the game continually changing, determining the true prevalence of autism (the number of cases in a specific population) is like trying to hit a moving target. But even statistical manipulation does not appear to fully explain the rising diagnosis rate.[13]

Characteristics of Autism

The medical definition of autism spectrum disorder is "a biologically based developmental disorder that is highly heritable."[14] Autism affects each person in a different manner, but generally it is characterized by impairments in social interaction, impairments in communication, restricted interests and repetitive behavior. Autism is four times more prevalent in boys than in girls.

Autism often appears initially as a noticeable language delay, which can be both in spoken language and comprehension and, for some children, a loss of previously acquired skills. Many parents report that early in their child's development they became concerned when the child fixated on objects, avoided eye contact, and engaged in hand flapping or other repetitive movements. Simple developmental stages, such as picking up language from the environment, imitating behavior or playing reciprocally may be delayed or absent. It can be difficult to assess a child's cognitive abilities because language impairments may make it impossible to accurately ascertain what he or she

12 Wazana, Bresnahan, & Kline (2007, pp. 721-730).
13 Newschaffer, Croen, & Daniels (2007, pp. 235-258).
14 Johnson, Myers, & CEC (2007).

truly comprehends, especially in the absence of language or in the presence of silent seizures.

Many children with autism exhibit a need for rigid routines and exhibit ritualistic behaviors and sensory disturbances. These children usually make little or no eye contact. Some children cry more than typically developing children, stiffen when held and appear quite happy to be left alone. Others exhibit communication problems such as echolalia (repeating what was just said to them) and pronoun reversal (for example, a child referring to himself as "he" or "you").

Behavioral disturbances can be seen at all stages of development; in some instances, they are severe and extremely violent. Children may injure themselves and others or display obsessive-compulsive-type behaviors, impulsiveness, mood swings and agitation. In some children, aggression and rage may manifest suddenly, often escalating during puberty. Some speculate that hormonal changes are behind the exacerbation of aggression seen at that time.[15]

Despite challenges and deficits, areas of strength, such as memory, are usually found as well. For example, an estimated 0.5 to 10 percent of individuals with ASD show unusual abilities, ranging from splinter skills such as memorization of trivia to the extraordinary and rare talents of prodigious savants.[16] Many children with autism have average to above-average intelligence and are very capable of learning, participating in community life, working and attending school, although they sometimes may need supportive services. In the highest functioning form of autism, a person may have superior and even genius intelligence. Others have a more obvious intellectual disability and may grow into adults who will need support and supervision.

---

15 Edelson (2005, p. 3).
16 Treffert (2009).

Characteristics of Autism Spectrum Disorders

- ASD affects each individual in a different manner but is generally characterized by impairments in social interactions and communication skills. In some people, it also affects cognitive, emotional and behavioral functioning. Individuals with Asperger Syndrome (also know as high-functioning autism) may have superior skills and intelligence.

- ASD is four times more prevalent in boys than in girls.

- No one is sure what causes ASD, but studies of twins reveal that it is potentially a genetically based condition. In identical twins, there is an 80-90 percent chance that each will have autism and in non-identical twins there is a 3-10 percent chance that both will develop it. The chance that siblings will be affected by autism is also approximately 3-10 percent.

- Early signs of ASD may include lack of social interaction, communication, and inappropriate behavior. Signs may be detected in infants as young as 6-18 months, and are often reported by parents who are concerned that their child fixates on objects, does not respond to his or her name, avoids eye contact and engages in repetitive movements such as rocking or arm flapping.

- In 2007, the Centers for Disease Control and Prevention's (CDC) Autism and Developmental Disabilities Monitoring Network determined that 1 in 150 children are diagnosed with autism in the United States. In some states the diagnosis is more prevalent.

- In 2012 the rate is said to be 1 in 88, according to the CDC. That is 1 in 54 boys.

- Autism is a lifelong challenge, and most, including those with Asperger Syndrome, will require some sort of support and services throughout their lifetime.

- Individuals with autism have diverse talents and abilities and can live, work and recreate in community settings with the proper support.

From http://www.djfiddlefoundation.org/. Used with permission.

Some Historical Facts About Autism[17]

The history of autism goes as far back as 1910 when Eugene Bleuler, a Swiss psychiatrist, first coined the term.[18]

- In 1943, Dr. Leo Kanner of Johns Hopkins University described early infantile autism for the first time,[19] basing his discovery on 11 children he observed between 1938 and 1943 who demonstrated striking behavioral similarities. Dr. Kanner coined the phrase "refrigerator mothers," referring to mothers who did not provide adequate emotional attention, to describe an apparent coldness he observed in many mothers of autistic children. He believed the sources of autism were innate in the affected child but that unemotional parental behavior exacerbated the problem. Almost all of the characteristics described in Kanner's first paper on the subject, notably "autistic aloneness" and "insistence on sameness," are regarded as typical of autism spectrum disorders.[20]

- During the 1940s and through the 1960s, the medical community felt that children who had autism where schizophrenic, psychotic or out of touch with reality.

- A school of thought advanced by Dr. Bruno Bettelheim, a widely known, self-promoting professor of child development in the 1940s-1970s, revived the "refrigerator mothers" idea, suggesting parents did not provide adequate emotional nurturing and even comparing parents to guards in Nazi concentration camps. The theory has since been completely discarded.[21]

---

17 Reynolds & Dombeck (2006).
18 *Autism history.* http://www.news-medical.net/health/Autism-History.aspx
19 Kanner (1943).
20 Happé, Ronald, & Plomin (2006).
21 *Refrigerator mothers.* (2006). http://autism.about.com/od/causesofautism/p/refrigerator.htm

- Currently, a new school of thought exists in support of a diathesis-stress mode of causation. This theory suggests that it takes two events to bring about an illness. Initially, a genetic vulnerability enhances susceptibility. Next, a stressful event or events, tied to the environment, acts as a catalyst.[22]

Is Autism a "Catch-All" Diagnosis?"

Perhaps the "spectrum" of behaviors and disturbances that we tend to lump together under the term *autism* is not a single disorder but a series of behaviors and challenges that have many different underlying conditions but share some common attributes, such as seizure and disturbances in language, socialization and responses to the environment.

There is no one single genetic or cognitive cause for the diverse symptoms that define autism.[23] Studies of twins diagnosed with autism suggest that it is potentially a genetically based disorder. Thus, there is an 80-90 percent chance that both identical twins will have autism if one of them does. The fraternal twin of an affected sibling has a 3-10 percent chance of developing autism. By comparison, the chance that typical siblings will both be affected is in the range of 3-10 percent. Further, chromosomal defects such as Rett syndrome, Fragile X syndrome and a genetic enzyme deficiency called phenylketonuria (PKU) greatly increase the chance a child will be diagnosed with autism. For more information, see Chapter 3.

At the same time, there is mounting evidence to suggest that genetic mutations (permanent change or damage in DNA) are at the root of many cases of autism. Thus, many genetic diseases greatly increase the chance that a child develops features similar to autism, since they produce very similar traits[24] (see Chapter 3).

---

22 Reynolds & Dombeck (2006).
23 Happé et al. (2006).
24 *Causes of autism*. http://en.wikipedia.org/wiki/Causes_of_autism

In 2011, a common genetic cause of autism and epilepsy was discovered. A research team, led by neurologist Dr. Patrick Cossette,
found a severe mutation (change in DNA, our hereditary material of
life) on the SYN1 gene in a family suffering from epilepsy, including
individuals who also had autism. For the first time, these results
show that the role of the SYN1 gene occurs in autism and epilepsy,
thus strengthening the hypothesis that a dysregulation of the function of the synapse (nerve cell) due to this severe genetic mutation
is the cause of both diseases.[25] (The synapse is the structure that
permits a nerve cell to pass an electrical signal to another cell.) Due
to the damage of this gene, the synapse cannot function properly,
leading to impairment of the organ function, in this case, the brain.

---

25 Cossette et al. (2011, pp. 2297-2307).

CHAPTER 3

COMMON GENETIC DISORDERS FOUND IN BOTH AUTISM AND EPILEPSY

Many disorders that are genetic in origin produce seizures along with a pervasive developmental disorder and, therefore, are of interest in this context. This chapter outlines some of the more prevalent genetic disorders that may be found in both autism and epilepsy.

While reading, please remember that accurate diagnosis requires careful observation of symptoms by the family/caregivers, appropriate communication with physicians and other professionals about those symptoms and careful evaluation of the patient by appropriately trained and experienced professionals using current testing methods.

Lennox-Gastaut

Epilepsy syndrome marked by numerous seizure types, including tonic, absence (including atypical) and atonic seizures. Additionally, regression along with intellectual impairment is seen. This syndrome is more common in boys than in girls. The possible etiologies (causes) are:

1. Prenatal, perinatal or postnatal lack of oxygen or brain infection

2. Congenital malformation of the brain

3. Disorders of the skin and nervous system

4. Metabolic disorders – deficiencies in the ability to enzymatically process chemicals in the body, such as abnormalities with the metabolism of amino acids, organic acids or mitochondrial function

5. Chromosomal disorders

6. Degenerative neurological disorders[26]

Angelman Syndrome

Shares a common genetic basis with some forms of autism. Characterized by deficits in cognition and language. Spoken language is often more of a problem than understanding language. Seizures frequently accompany this disorder. [27] Autism is commonly diagnosed in individuals with Angelman Syndrome.[28]

Childhood Disintegrative Disorder, or CDD

Rare form of autism with a strong male preponderance.[29] Symptoms may appear by age 2, but the average onset is between 3 and 4 years of age. Until that time, the child has age-appropriate skills in communication and social relationships. The loss of skills such as vocabulary are more dramatic in CDD than in other forms of autism. (The long period of normal development sets this apart from Rett Syndrome.) The diagnosis requires extensive and pronounced losses involving motor, language and social skills. CDD is also often accompanied by seizures.[30]

---

26 Kutscher (2006, p. 129).
27 Guerrini, Carrozzo, Rinaldi, & Bonanni (2003).
28 Philpot, Mabb, & Judson (2011). http://sfari.org/news-and-opinion/viewpoint/2011/insights-for-autism-from-angelman-syndrome
29 Frombonne (2002, pp. 149-157).
30 Frombonne (2002).

Landau-Kleffner Syndrome

Childhood disorder characterized by a progressive loss of the ability to understand and use spoken language (aphasia). The disorder typically appears in children between ages 3 and 7 years old who are otherwise developing normally. The seizure component of this condition is so strong that it is often called *acquired epileptic aphasia* or *aphasia with convulsive disorder*. Because the seizures tend to occur at night, the condition may be diagnosed through a sleep EEG. Language recovery is often possible with treatment, which includes antiseizure medications and steroids.[31] Most children with Laundau-Kleffner Syndrome have impaired intellectual functioning and/or information processing and developmental delays.[32] (See also pp. 127-129.)

Progressive Myoclonic Epilepsies

Rare form of epilepsy frequently resulting from hereditary metabolic disorders. They feature a combination of myoclonic and tonic-clonic seizures. Unsteadiness, muscle rigidity and mental deterioration are often also present. They grow progressively worse over time and often become resistant to antiseizure medications.[33]

Isodicentric 15 (abbreviated as idic 15)

Caused by mutations in chromosome 15 and associated with certain physical characteristics such as distinct facial features, low muscle tone and short stature. Anxiety disorders, attention deficit disorders, autism spectrum disorders and seizures are commonly seen in children with idic 15.[34]

---

31 Volkmar & Rutter (1995, pp. 1092-1095).
32 Landau-Kleffner Syndrome. http://www.ninds.nih.gov/disorders/landaukleffnersyndrome/landaukleffnersyndrome.htm
33 *Progressive myoclonic epilepsies*. http://www.epilepsy.com/epilepsy/epilepsy_promyoclonic
34 Battaglia, Parrini, & Tancredi (2010).

Rett Syndrome

Caused by mutations in a gene located on the X chromosome and seen more commonly in girls. Children with Rett Syndrome may develop typically at first and then begin to regress after about 18 months, hence its association and often confusion with autism. In fact, Rett Syndrome has been called "the most common basis of autism in girls."[35] The syndrome slows growth of the head and the brain as well as hands and feet. Features include repetitive hand movements, learning disabilities, problems with socialization and slowed or absent verbal skills. The *Diagnostic and Statistical Manual of Mental Disorders, Fourth Edition* (DSM-IV) classifies Rett Syndrome as a pervasive developmental disorder.[36]

Fragile X Syndrome

Also a mutation of the X chromosome. This genetic disorder, also an inherited form of impaired intellectual function, is more commonly expressed in boys. Distinctive features include a long face, prominent ears and hyper-extendable joints. Like Rett Syndrome, Fragile X overlaps with the autism spectrum and has been called "the most common genetic cause of autism."[37]

Soto Syndrome

Rare genetic disorder in which children grow excessively during their first few years. Children with Soto Syndrome have long, narrow heads with a facial appearance characterized by increased space between the eyes, a protruding forehead and a pointed chin. These patients have cognitive deficits (mild intellectual impairment) and speech impairments, and thus this disorder may be mistaken for (or considered a genetic cause of) autism. In addition, those with

---

35 Tropea et al. (2009, pp. 2029-2034).
36 *Rett syndrome*. http://en.wikipedia.org/wiki/Rett_syndrome
37 Fragile X. http://www.fraxa.org

Soto Syndrome may exhibit attention deficit hyperactivity disorder (ADHD), phobias, obsessive/compulsive behaviors, tantrums, impulsive behavior and unusual aggressiveness or irritability.[38]

Tuberous Sclerosis Complex

Genetic disorder that causes growth of nonmalignant tumors in organs such as the brain, eyes, heart, kidney, skin and lungs. Mild cases may produce few noticeable mental or behavioral problems. About half to two thirds of people with tuberous sclerosis have a developmental delay that can range from mild learning disabilities to severe intellectual impairment, according to the National Institute of Neurological Disorders and Stroke (NINDS).[39]

Neurofibromatosis Type 1

Neurologic disease with genetic causes that frequently overlap with autism. The condition causes tumors called neurofibromas and can sometimes be diagnosed through the characteristic light brown skin patches called café-au-lait spots. While the common ground between the two conditions is unknown, patients diagnosed with autism have over 100 times the risk of having neurofibromatosis, which suggests a common underlying cause.[40]

Moebius Syndrome

Results in loss of the function of the cranial nerves, which prevents a person from making normal facial expressions, such as smiling and eye movement. Some people with this condition appear typical in social development and intellect. However, about 10 percent have intellectual impairment. In one study of people with Moebius Syndrome, 40 percent demonstrated symptoms typical of autism. The

38 Soto syndrome. http://www.ninds.nih.gov/disorders/sotos/sotos.htm
39 Soto syndrome. http://www.ninds.nih.gov/disorders/sotos/sotos.htm
40 *Genetics overview*. www.exploringautism.org

study's authors suggest that this may be due to a "common under-lying neurobiological deficit at the brainstem level."[41]

Smith-Magenis Syndrome

Traced to chromosome 17, this is another genetic abnormality with behavioral characteristics similar to autism. People with this syndrome are usually affectionate and engaging but may have be-havioral problems, such as frequent tantrums or outbursts, aggres-sion, anxiety, impulsiveness and attention deficits. Behavioral traits include self-injury (biting, hitting, head banging and skin picking) and also traits somewhat unique to this condition such as repetitive self-hugging and a tendency to lick fingers while flipping the pages of books and magazines.[42]

Rubenstein-Taybi Syndrome

Caused by mutations in a gene-binding protein. Distinctive facial features accompany this disorder along with broad thumbs and toes, excess weight, short stature and poor muscle coordination. The disorder is characterized by impaired intellectual function and behavior problems such as a short attention span and a tendency toward repetitive movements.[43]

West Syndrome

Also called infantile spasms, this is a rare seizure disorder that causes developmental disabilities and traits similar to those seen in autism, including intellectual disability and behavior issues. This syndrome produces a pattern often detectable on EEG.[44]

---

41 Gillberg & Billstedt (2000, pp. 321-330).
42 Smith-Magenis syndrome. http://www.ncbi.nlm.nih.gov/books/NBK1310/
43 Rubenstein-Taybi syndrome. http://www.ncbi.nlm.nih.gov/pubmed/7630403
44 About epilepsy. http://www.epilepsyfoundation.org/about/types/ syndromes/infantilespasms.cfm

Fetal Alcohol Syndrome

Caused by a maternal alcohol use during pregnancy. It produces a set of symptoms similar to those seen in autism, specifically social skill deficits and speech delays. It is completely preventable by not drinking alcohol while pregnant.[45]

Phenylketonuria (PKU)

Caused by lack of an essential amino acid, thus creating a deficiency that interferes with protein metabolism.[46] PKU can cause seizures along with intellectual disability that mimic the features seen in autism.

Purine Disorders

Associated with purines, which are chemicals needed to sustain life. Some give us energy and aid in the metabolism of food. There are many different purine disorders, each producing a genetic syndrome that often includes an autistic presentation with a seizure component, in addition to other issues.[47]

Rubella

Caused by the virus that causes German measles. It causes damage to a developing fetus in utero.[48] One proposed etiology for autism is viral infection very early in development. The mechanism by which viral infection may lead to autism is not known, be it through direct infection of the central nervous system (CNS) or through infection elsewhere in the body acting as a trigger for disease in the CNS, through alteration of the immune response of the mother or offspring, or a combination of these. The best association to date

---

45 *Fetal alcohol syndrome.* http://www.ncbi.nlm.nih.gov/pubmedhealth/PMH0001909/
46 *What is autism?* http://www.acesautism.com/faq.html
47 Nyhan (2005).
48 *Definition of fetal rubella effects.* http://www.medterms.com/script/main/art.asp?articlekey=16130

has been made between congenital rubella and autism; however, members of the herpes virus family may also play a role in autism.[49]

Lactic Acidosis

A buildup of toxins in the blood; occurs with many inborn errors of metabolism as a syndrome resembling autism and can be a manifestation of ASD. In a research study,[50] four patients were found to have two coexistent syndromes: the behavioral syndrome of autism and the biochemical syndrome of lactic acidosis. These findings raise the possibility that one subgroup of the autism syndrome is associated with inborn errors of carbohydrate metabolism.

> As mentioned at the beginning of this chapter, it is essential that family and caregivers seek out the appropriate medical professionals who can help determine if any of these syndromes exist, and thus the correct treatment.

Evidence for the Seizure-Autism Connection

According to Dr. Bryan King, director of child and adolescent psychiatry at Seattle Children's Hospital, "as many as 40 percent of children and young adults with autism may experience seizure."[51] Further, adolescence is a time of particular vulnerability to seizures in these children.

The percentage quoted by Dr. King may actually underestimate the problem, since partial seizures (those affecting only a small part of one hemisphere of the brain) often elude detection, and thus go undiagnosed.[52]

---

49 Libbey, Sweeten, McMahon, & Fujinami (2005).
50 Coleman & Blass (1985).
51 Marikar, Childs, & Chitale (2009).
52 N. Minshew (personal communication, June 4, 2008).

Researchers Munoz-Yunta et al. speculate that 20 percent of children with the diagnosis of autism suffer from some kind of epileptic seizures, and another 80 percent suffer from the subclinical variety. (The symptoms of seizure are so subtle that they are not easily detected, and thus they are not manifested or clinically evident by conventional methods currently employed.)[53]

In another line of research, Dr. Holmes Morton, a Harvard-trained physician who is well known for his work in studying genetic diseases in the Amish and Mennonite populations of Pennsylvania, discovered a mutation on a gene[54] associated with focal epilepsy syndrome (in which seizures occur in a small part of the brain rather than the entire brain – also known as partial epilepsy). Through a simple blood test, this condition, known as cortical focal epilepsy syndrome, can now be identified at birth.

According to Dr. Morton, evidence suggests that focal epilepsy syndrome produces traits similar to those seen in autism. In fact, he notes that some of his patients with a presentation of autism also experience partial seizures and that these seizures cause some of the symptoms that lead to the diagnosis of autism.

In interviews, Dr. Morton reported that when he has referred some of his "seizing" patients to neurologists, he has had to convince these nuerologists that the patients were having silent seizures. Thus, many physicians still hold the belief that a positive EEG result is required to confirm a diagnosis of epilepsy, and without it, are reluctant to diagnose or treat seizures.[55]

---

53 Munoz-Yunta et al. (2003).
54 H. Morton (personal communication, June 18, 2007).
55 N. Minshew (personal communication, June 4, 2008).

Evidence of Cause?

A Canadian researcher and physician Angela Gedye[56] asked an important question: Can seizures actually be causing autism and not merely be casually associated with the diagnosis? She noted that many of the behaviors we see in people with autism, such as staring and screaming, are also common in frontal lobe seizures. Is it merely a coincidence that these frontal lobe seizures are known to produce screaming, rage, aggression and self-injury?

Gedye suggests that certain involuntary movements such as scratching, slapping, spitting, skin picking and punching oneself in the head often occur during seizures. Abnormal electrical discharges in the brain produced by the seizure can result in these rigid muscle contractions and uncontrolled movements.

Current theories regarding causes of self-injurious behavior range from attention seeking to frustration with communication limitations. However, Gedye is skeptical of these interpretations, noting that people with Tourette Syndrome, who have normal intelligence and severe self-injurious involuntary movements, for example, do not perform these types of actions to gain attention or in response to frustration with communication. Instead, they often ask for help in preventing these behaviors, clearly indicating that the behaviors are involuntary.[57]

How Can It Be That the Seizures in Certain Autistic Brains Are Overlooked?

As regrettable and unacceptable as this is, it is not totally surprising that seizures in individuals with autism are often overlooked.

---

56 Gedye (1991, pp. 174-182).
57 Gedye (1991, pp. 174-182).

First, consider the unusual behavior seen with these seizures that make them look psychiatric in nature. For example, a person mumbling incoherently who then begins to complain of either seeing visions or hearing voices could so easily be misdiagnosed as suffering a psychiatric illness. Interestingly, these partial seizures go undiagnosed in as many as half of the patients who suffer from them, even those who appear to have typical intellectual development, according to Eve LaPlante, who wrote the book *Seized*[58] (see Chapter 5). Also consider the multiple barriers to diagnosis in individuals with autism (for example, they may be unable to describe what they are experiencing or unable to engage in conversation with unfamiliar people, such as medical specialists). On top of those hurdles, the test used to discover these deep seizures (a surface routine scalp EEG) often misses the electrical storm and is read as normal.

Dr. Nancy Minshew, an internationally recognized autism expert and director of the Center for Excellence in Autism Research at the University of Pittsburgh, explains that some seizures originate so deep in the brain's temporal lobe (see Chapter 4) that the electricity they generate is not measurable on a standard EEG. Dr. Minshew agrees that if this "electrical storm" is not occurring while the EGG test is being performed, it will go undetected. She goes so far as to say that a person could have many EEGs with normal results and still harbor an undetected seizure disorder.[59] Despite the absence of EEG findings, seizures often exist. As a result, the diagnosis must be made by astute observation and recording of symptoms over time.

With so many possible sources of autism to consider, and with precious time for implementing therapies ticking away, families are eager to discover what is happening and then settle upon the appropriate therapy.

58 LaPlante (1993, 2000).
59 N. Minshew (personal communication, June 4, 2008).

CHAPTER 4

WHAT ARE BRAIN SEIZURES?

What could be more complicated and mysterious than the human brain? This big gob of grey material encased in bone controls everything we do. It guides our thoughts and dreams, organizes our reality, directs our behavior, movement, and breathing, and controls our senses of sight, hearing, smell and touch, as well as the sometimes mysterious, enigmatic emotions we experience. The brain is the seat of our memory.

The typical brain is complicated and mysterious, and autism and the seizures that often co-exist deepen the mystery, showing us what can happen when the brain has a varied and altered course.

Autism and Seizures

In 2008, the Centers for Disease Control and Prevention (CDC) reported that 2.7 million Americans have epilepsy and that epilepsy affects 1 in 100 adults.[60] Autism and epilepsy occur together in one third of people diagnosed with autism.[61] The co-existence of autism and epilepsy is well documented when we talk about the generalized tonic-clonic seizure type better known as grand mal. This occurs when the whole brain is involved and a person falls to the ground and convulses.

Partial seizures do not involve the entire brain and do not cause falling. These invisible seizures can co-exist with autism too but are

60 Aetna (n.d.).
61 Gabis, Pomeroy, & Andriola (2005).

hard to detect, which deepens the mystery and adds to the complicated array of behaviors we see accompanying this condition.

A "seizure" is an abnormal electrical discharge that originates inside of the brain and then causes a behavioral change. The type of seizure depends upon the area of the brain where the discharge originated.

It is important to note that **not all seizures signify an epilepsy diagnosis**. A person can have an isolated event of seizure, such as in connection with a high fever or brain tumor. Epilepsy, on the other hand, is as a tendency toward recurring seizures that are unprovoked by any systemic or acute neurologic problem. Traditionally, the diagnosis of epilepsy requires the occurrence of at least two unprovoked seizures 24 hours apart.

"Visualize the brain as a coordinated network of electrical discharges and signals," suggests Dr. Minshew. "During these seizures there is chaos in communication, and the signals degenerate. This in turn causes thinking and behavior to deteriorate. If a small area of the brain is affected, it may be noticed only in lesser, more subtle oddities. Conversely, if a larger area is affected, a more involved scenario unfolds. This makes sense when we break it down and examine it. We need to become familiar with the sneaky, "stealth," subclinical way these smaller electrical malfunctions manifest inside our children's brains."

Dr. Minshew further explains, "The brain is complicated, with many different parts, which is not unlike looking under the hood of a car. If our car breaks down, we immediately look under the hood to see what it could be. We look closely at the parts individually, since each part has a job and a function to carry out, and together the parts make the car run optimally. It is the same with seizures and autism. It takes a superb brain mechanic who is highly trained to identify the brain problems at their root."[62] We must take a closer look at the brains of every child diagnosed with autism.

Basic Brain Anatomy

Here's a very simple overview of the human brain. The cerebrum, or cortex, is the largest part of the brain. It is made up of two halves, the right and left hemispheres. These halves are connected by long neuron branches. The left side of the brain controls the right side of the body and vice versa. Each hemisphere, in turn, is made up of four lobes or sections: the frontal, occipital, parietal and temporal lobe. Each lobe is responsible for various functions within the body, as illustrated below.

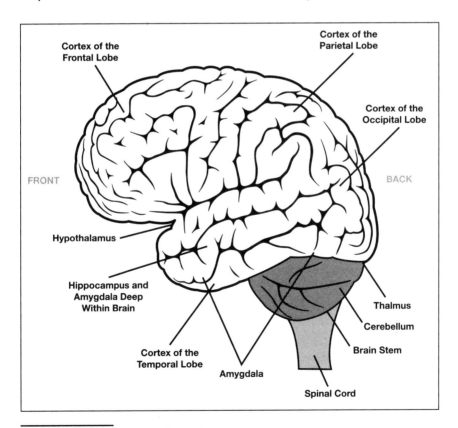

---

62 N. Minshew (personal communication, June 4, 2008).

Frontal lobe: Lying behind the forehead, this lobe controls our reasoning, conscious thought, learning, speech, personality and voluntary movement.

Temporal lobe: Located just above the ears, this lobe is responsible for our emotions, memory, speech, and hearing and how we view the world around us.

Parietal lobe: Located behind the frontal lobe, this lobe controls how we feel and process sensory information, how we judge spatial relationships, movement and our coordination.

Occipital lobe: Located at the back of the brain just behind the parietal lobe, this lobe assists us in gathering information from our eyes and making sense of the world around us.

The cerebellum: Lying under the hemispheres, this helps to coordinate all the areas of the brain so they can work together. Thus, it plays an important role in balance and movement.

The brain stem: This is the part of the brain that connects to the spinal cord and controls our breathing and heartbeat.

The hippocampus: Located in the mid-brain as part of the temporal lobe, this is the part that assists us in learning and forming memories.

The amygdala: Located in the cerebrum, it is an important component of the neural network that underlies social behavior. It is alert to the needs of basic survival and is also involved in emotional reactions such as anger and fear. Studies of autistic brains at autopsy have identified abnormalities in this part of the brain. It is believed that autism affects the amygdala, cerebellum, and many other parts of the brain.[63]

---

63 Amaral, Schumann, & Nordahl (2008).

Hypothalamus: Located at the base of the brain where signals from the brain and the body's hormonal system interact and maintain the body's status quo. The hypothalamus monitors such things as blood pressure and body temperature.

Thalmus: Located on the top of the brain stem, it is thought of as a two-way relay station directing signals from the spinal cord up to the cerebrum and, conversely, from the cerebrum down to the spinal cord and nervous system.

Seizures and the Brain

Let's look more closely at seizures, their origin and nature, and the areas they may affect.

The temporal lobe is the most vulnerable lobe in the brain to epileptic discharges, and most often this is where a seizure originates. Temporal lobe epilepsy (TLE), or absence seizure, is a brain disorder that occurs when there is sudden abnormal electrical discharge from deep inside the brain, which causes behavior changes. The two types of seizures associated with TLE are the simple partial (awareness intact) and complex partial (loss of awareness). If the seizure spreads to involve both temporal lobes, memory will be affected. Occasionally, as a result of the spreading to both brain lobes, the complex partial seizure becomes generalized or – a tonic-clonic seizure – with a loss of consciousness and violent muscle contractions. This is what most people imagine when they think of a seizure.[64] Unfortunately, for many sufferers of partial seizures, this stereotypical view of a seizure may lead to a lack of diagnosis and treatment (see Chapter 6).

Many seizure types are known to co-exist with autism. The following is a list of the most common (see Chapter 5 for further information about each).

---

64 *Depression.* http://www.mayoclinic.com/health/grand-mal-seizure/DS00222

Types of Seizures

Autism, Epilepsy & Seizures: How to Recognize the Signs and Basic First Aid When You Do

SEIZURE TYPE	WHAT IT LOOKS LIKE	WHAT IT IS NOT	WHAT TO DO	WHAT NOT TO DO
Generalized Tonic Clonic (Also called Grand Mal)	Sudden cry, fall, rigidity, followed by muscle jerks, shallow breathing or temporarily suspended breathing, bluish skin, possible loss of bladder or bowel control, usually lasts a couple of minutes. Normal breathing then starts again. There may be some confusion and/or fatigue, followed by return to full consciousness.	Heart attack. Stroke.	Look for medical identification. Protect from nearby hazards. Loosen tie or shirt collar. Protect head from injury. Turn on side to keep airway clear unless injury exists. Reassure as consciousness returns. If single seizure lasted less than 5 minutes, ask if hospital evaluation wanted. If multiple seizures, or if one seizure lasts longer than 5 minutes, call an ambulance. If person is pregnant, injured, or diabetic, call for aid at once.	Don't put anything in the mouth. Don't try to hold tongue. It can't be swallowed. Don't try to give liquids during or just after seizure. Don't use artificial respiration unless breathing is absent after muscle jerks subside. Don't restrain.
Absence (Also called Petit Mal)	A blank stare, beginning and ending abruptly, lasting only a few seconds, most common in children. May be accompanied by rapid blinking, some chewing movements of the mouth. Child or adult is unaware of what's going on during the seizure, but quickly returns to full awareness once it has stopped. May result in learning difficulties if not recognized and treated.	Daydreaming. Lack of attention. Deliberately ignoring adult instructions.	No first aid necessary, but if this is the first observation of a seizure, medical evaluation is recommended.	
Simple Partial	Jerking may begin in one area of body, arm, leg, or face. Can't be stopped, but patient stays awake and aware. Jerking may proceed from one area of the body to another, and sometimes spreads to become a generalized convulsive seizure.	Acting out, bizarre behavior. Hysteria. Mental illness. Psychosomatic illness. Parapsychological or mystical experience.	No first aid necessary unless seizure becomes convulsive, then first aid as above. No immediate action needed other than reassurance and emotional support. Medical evaluation is recommended.	

SEIZURE TYPE	WHAT IT LOOKS LIKE	WHAT IT IS NOT	WHAT TO DO	WHAT NOT TO DO
Complex Partial (Also called Psychomotor or Temporal Lobe)	Usually starts with blank stare, followed by chewing, followed by random activity. Person appears unaware of surroundings, may seem dazed and mumble. Unresponsive. Actions clumsy, not directed. May pick at clothing, pick up objects, try to take clothes off. May run, appear afraid. May struggle or flail at restraint. Once pattern established, same set of actions usually occur with each seizure. Lasts a few minutes, but post-seizure confusion can last substantially longer. No memory of what happened during seizure period.	Drunkenness. Intoxication from drugs. Mental illness. Disorderly conduct.	Speak calmly and reassuringly to patient and others. Guide gently away from obvious hazards. Stay with person until completely aware of environment. Offer help getting home.	Don't grab hold unless sudden danger (such as a cliff edge or an approaching car) threatens. Don't try to restrain. Don't shout. Don't expect verbal response.
Atonic Seizures (Also called Drop Attacks)	A child or adult suddenly collapses and falls. After 10 seconds to a minute he recovers, regains consciousness, and can stand and walk again.	Clumsiness. Normal childhood "stage." In a child, lack of good walking skills. In an adult, drunkenness, acute illness.	No first aid needed, unless the person was hurt upon falling. Medical evaluation is recommended.	
Myoclonic Seizures	Sudden brief, massive muscle jerks that may involve the whole body or parts of the body. May cause person to spill what they were holding or fall off a chair.	Clumsiness Poor coordination.	No first aid needed, but medical evaluation is recommended.	
Infantile Spasms	These are clusters of quick, sudden movements that start between 3 months and two years. If a child is sitting up, the head will fall forward, and the arms will flex forward. If lying down, the knees will be drawn up, with arms and bead flexed forward as if the baby is reaching for support.	Normal movements of the baby. Colic.	No first aid needed, but medical evaluation is recommended.	

From http://www.djfiddlefoundation.org/. Used with permission.

Where in the Brain Do Seizures Originate?

Temporal lobe: As noted above, the partial epilepsies origi-nate in the temporal lobe of the brain. They can be classified into two sub-types; **Mesial temporal lobe** epilepsy, in which the aura is defined by stomach upset or mouth movements. **Lateral temporal lobe** epilepsy is often accompanied by au-ditory (hearing) or visual (seeing) hallucinations, illusions and body rotation.

Frontal lobe: A large spectrum of seizure can originate from the frontal lobe, including simple partial, complex partial, tonic-clonic, atonic and myoclonic. These seizures tend to begin quickly, last briefly and end quickly.

Parietal lobe: The parietal lobes are located behind the frontal lobes and are involved in the processing of sensations. Nota-ble are the sensations produced such as pins and needles, pain and disturbances of smell or vision.

Occipital lobe: The occipital lobe primarily controls our vision. These seizures produce disturbance of sight such as seeing col-ored lights or black dots or temporary visual loss. Diversion of the head may be seen along with eye blinking or eye shaking.

Partial Seizures

We will take a closer look at partial seizures as these are most relevant to this discussion. There are two types of partial seizures: simple and complex.

A **simple partial seizure** does not affect consciousness. However, movement, emotions, sensations and behavior may be affected. Some people having a simple partial seizure are fully aware but cannot respond for the duration of the seizure. A person can usu-ally remember it afterward, and it might look something like this:

Movement: Uncontrollable movements in any part of the body. Eyes may move from side to side, and there may be blinking, unusual movements of the mouth or tongue and twitching of the face. It may start with shaking of a foot and move on to one whole side of the body.

Emotions: A sudden feeling of fear or a sense that something terrible is about to occur may ensue. The individual may experience sudden joy or sorrow, uncontrollable laughing, screaming or a sudden burst of rage and anger.

Senses: Any or all the senses can be involved. A seizure can produce the hallucinated feeling of a breeze to the skin, the perception of a smell from something burning or seeing things that are not really there. These distortions seem very real to those who are experiencing it.

A **complex partial seizure** alters consciousness, either impairing it or making a person lose it, so the person cannot interact with others successfully. These seizures affect a larger area of the brain. During a complex partial seizure, the person has no idea what she is doing and does not remember it later. It has been characterized as a seizure "standing up." That is, the person is in a deep trance-like state and looks significantly impaired. It is an altered state of consciousness, and even though the person's eyes are open and she may say things, she has no idea what she is doing, and any speech is garbled or gibberish rather than purposeful language. It is a dreamlike state similar to sleepwalking.

Typically, a complex partial seizure begins with a blank stare and loss of contact with surroundings, followed by alterations in the seven senses. Screaming, chewing, picking or fumbling with clothes may occur, and the person may exhibit disorganized motor movements such as flailing the arms or bicycling with the legs, sometimes even undressing. The person may run, cry out and repeat the same phrase over and over. Some people become violent and aggressive, but usually such behavior is unfocused and undirected and can be minimized by trying not to restrain. Sometimes the person bites down on the skin with clenched teeth and hurts himself or others with random acts of aggression.

How Seizures Damage the Brain

According to Dr. Holmes' paper "Effects of Seizures on Brain Development: Lessons From the Laboratory," recurring seizures may contribute to nerve cell injury in the developing brain and may be associated with a decline in cognitive function. Seizures have been induced in laboratory animals, and subsequent brain changes were measured. Computer statistical analysis was done to ascertain if the volume of nerve cells had changed after the seizures occurred with electrical stimulation. The conclusion was that certain populations of nerve cells may die after a single and/or repeated seizure. Molecular signals inside the nerve cells of the brain led to their death. The studies also concluded that some genes can either protect the brain or make it more susceptible to injury after seizures.

Researchers have noted that seizures can alter brains in other ways besides nerve cell death. Rewiring of the brain's complex circuitry and the birth of newer brain cells both may be contributory. The extent of the impact upon a specific brain may depend on the age at which these seizures begin. Both clinical and lab studies demonstrate that seizures early in life can result in permanent behavioral abnormalities and enhance the chance of epilepsy.[65] Therefore, as repeated throughout this book, these seizures must be recognized and treated as early as possible.

Temporal lobe epilepsy often occurs in the language hemisphere of the brain, producing severe delays in the processing of language and information. **Rolandic epilepsy**, previously considered to be a benign condition, has been revealed by recent studies to cause neu-

---

65 Holmes (2005, pp. 1-11).

rological deficits that impede learning and produce severe language delays. We are documenting numerous "mile markers" for children who appear to have a communication disorder but whose social interaction remains intact.[66]

What Does a Seizure Feel Like?

Josh is staring and has a faraway look in his eyes. Sometimes he complains about Sammy (a boy he knew years before who he says visits him during the hallucination of a seizure), and sometimes it's the one-eyed monster or Ninjas who intrude.

"Sammy is bothering me."

This is his vision that often recurs when he has a seizure. Though the experience occurred long ago, it makes him feel as if it is happening again.

"Leave me alone, you idiot!" he screams.

It is easy for a lay person to think this is the perseverative behavior (behavior that occurs over and over again) frequently seen in persons diagnosed with autism. Most parents have been told that this is a feature of autism and that we should simply expect to see it. Therefore, we often fail to realize it is a treatable component that may be produced by a *subclinical* seizure disorder – a disorder that cannot be identified in a clinical setting, such as the "hidden" seizures we are discussing here.

---

66 F. Miranda (personal communication, June 4, 2008).

If the behavior is a random outburst with no apparent provocation, we must ask ourselves, "Why would he be acting out this way? If it isn't in response to wanting something, then what is the point of the behavior?" The point is that there may *be* no point, because the behavior is completely out of the person's control.

Moments ago he was laughing and watching his favorite show on television. Now he appears to be possessed by demons. *What happened?* It is natural for caregivers to ask these questions, and to even get upset with the seizing person, or worse, place blame and express anger towards him because they believe the behavior is within one's control.

Daniel Tammet, a man diagnosed with autism and savant syndrome, but more widely known for using his incredible memory to recall the mathematical constant Pi (3.141...) to more than 22,500 decimal places, wrote in his biography *Born on a Blue Day* about the severity of his seizures. He describes a feeling of the room around him pulling away and the light inside it leaking out, as if time itself had coagulated and stretched out into a single lingering moment. He had no idea that he was having an epileptic seizure.[67]

Donna Williams, famous for her writings on living with autism (*Nobody Nowhere; Somebody Somewhere*), was formally diagnosed with autism and seizures. Donna shares some of the school's notes about her that she found at her mother's home.

Donna's teachers wrote, "She can't see things in front of her ... used to be a good student, now she's saying she can't read ... makes strange noises ... seems disoriented at times ... walks around in circles ... unaware of time and place."

---

67 Tammet (2007, p. 29).

Donna also shares in her blog (www.blog.donnawilliams.net) that initially her seizures were mistaken for psychosis because they involved altered consciousness, and as a result she was placed on the wrong class of medication. She was diagnosed with atypical epilepsy and suffers from several different types of seizure. (Epilepsy runs on her father's side of the family.) She tells us of staring spells, eye blinking and mental static. Her epilepsy was formally diagnosed after she experienced what she calls fugues. Fugues involved walking and not feeling quite conscious.

I would be somewhere between asleep and awake, but not sure which one it was. I call it a 'fugue' or a pathological amnesiac condition during which one is apparently conscious of one's actions but has no recollection of them after returning back to a normal state. I felt disoriented and a sense of internal panic, as if I were dreaming that I was in trouble but I was definitely awake. I would wander in the street in search of something vague. Then after, I would fade back into consciousness feeling very distressed, as if a stranger led me to the middle of nowhere and then woke me up.

I had other similar episodes, and I recall feeling as if I were being overtaken by feeling very odd and dreamy. The streets were turned around, leaving me feeling distressed and disoriented. My sense of direction was altered and I had no idea where my car was since the streets had changed, or so it seemed. Imagine that your brain suddenly starts to tilt and you cannot tell if you have shifted or it is the earth that has shifted.

I also have had earthquakes ... which are like physical hallucinations. I would be walking in my house and suddenly it seemed as if the whole house was violently shaking and making my whole body jerk terribly. I remained partially conscious of it and thus did not fall.

Some types of colored lights or repetitive sounds could trigger a sudden mania where I would feel tingling, and all visual and verbal meaning would disintegrate as my body lost its consciousness and I found myself squealing. I was very agitated, self-injurious, and completely disoriented because I could not recognize my surroundings or even my own hand. I remember feeling that every time these fugues would occur; it seemed I was being sucked into the big black nothingness, which seemed to be eating away at my soul. I didn't see my body parts as mine, so when they followed me, I tried to flee from them, actually ripping my skin as my body followed me. I realize this sounds bizarre.

Most episodes lasted 20 minutes and would begin with an aura comprised of tingling, excitability, and the progressive loss of meaning, followed by an acute phase that was only a few seconds and then fading between disorientation and distress and then an awakening. That one 'dreamy' part is a good feeling actually almost as if I was mildly stoned and it was peaceful. But often to experience a sudden stripping away of your mind and the loss of the ability to make sense of this world feels so distressing.[68]

Imagine experiencing this while others are pursuing you, trying to make you to think, respond and do things? It is quite understandable why a person on the autism spectrum who is besieged by seizures would exhibit the unusual behaviors that we, sometimes wrongly, deem "autistic."

68 http://blog.donnawilliams.net/2010/01/10/my-experiences-with-atypical-epilepsy/

The Story of "Little C"

The following was told by Dr. Ramanujapuram Anand, clinical director, Department of Neurology and Neurosurgery, I. P. Pavlov Medical University:[69]

I met little C for the first time in the follow-up clinic with his mother. He was 7 years old but looked much younger. He was well dressed and groomed, with bright eyes, short fair hair, and was shorter than the average child of that age. He walked into the room, making no eye contact.

He took a blank sheet of paper that lay on the desk and brought it over to a smaller table that stood in one corner of the room and started drawing. He had a sad and blank expression on his face with no reciprocal interaction and never spoke a word all through the session, which lasted nearly two hours. He seemed to be in his own world engrossed in his drawing, oblivious to the happenings in the room. By the end of the session, he had filled the page with figures of little trees in neat rows and columns that looked uncannily identical. His mother pointed out that this had pretty much been the routine in every follow-up clinic for the last two years.

C was born full-term after a normal pregnancy and was delivered normally. As far as the mother could remember, his early motor developmental milestones were normally achieved, but he was late to develop speech. He would have some restless nights when he tossed and turned in bed. He was a very easy child to look after as he was not at all demanding. He had no problems feeding and was adequately toilet trained. He was fully immunized. One day when he was around 2 years of age,

---

69 Anand (2005).

while his mother was feeding him, C suddenly "went blank" with a vacant stare and started making clicking noises with his tongue, which lasted for less than a minute. This did not recur, so the mother never consulted a doctor.

As he grew older, clear changes appeared in his behavior. He liked routines very much, and the slightest change would bring on a tantrum in which he would become quite aggressive. These were frequent, with violence mostly directed toward objects but sometimes toward his mother and siblings. By contrast, he was unusually caring toward the pet cat, and they seemed to like each other's company. He could indicate his needs but was less verbal than previously, and was very literal in the use of language. He preferred playing alone for long hours and never mixed with his siblings, a brother three years older and a sister one year younger. His play was unimaginative and repetitive. He had a fascination with trees. He liked to look at pictures of trees in books again and again. He liked drawing only pictures of trees.

From the age of 5, very often and very suddenly, he demonstrated behavior that was out of character for him. His eyes would suddenly appear glazed and his face would become pale. He would then make strange clicking noises with his tongue and repeated movements in the air as if trying to climb. This would last from a few seconds to several minutes. He would then sleep for several hours.

A maternal uncle had a learning disability. His mother had separated from his father when C was about one and a half years old, and there was no contact with the dad. The father had a history of violent behavior and was seeing a psychiatrist, but further details were not available. No problems with the siblings were reported. Mother, who had a high school educa-

tion, was unemployed. The family received emotional support from Mother's mother and sister.

C had been fully assessed by a child psychiatrist, a pediatrician, a child neurologist, a speech-language therapist and a clinical psychologist. He had undergone general physical and neurological examinations. His laboratory investigations included routine blood and urine analysis and genetic testing, which did not reveal any abnormalities. Psychometric tests reported a below-average intelligence in the borderline range. Routine and sleep EEGs showed paroxysmal abnormalities over the left temporal lobe. Results of an MRI scan of the brain were normal.

From the history, C demonstrates a qualitative impairment in the development of reciprocal social interaction and communication. It appears that this was evident from infancy, though in a subtle form. At 2 years of age, he appears to have had an absence seizure. Whether this contributed to causing further impairments or the progress was natural is hard to tell. He shows some restriction and repetition in his interests and activities. Speech was late to develop, but he was able to use it, though only in a concrete way. These features are consistent with a diagnosis of autism.

At the age of 5, he started having clear-cut seizures. Whether the behavioral difficulties were subtle forms of seizures is hard to tell. EEG revealed abnormalities with a left temporal lobe focus. These are consistent with a diagnosis of complex partial seizures.

C was receiving the antiepileptic medication Valproic acid, also called Depakote. He was identified as having special educational needs and was receiving specialized help in school. His mother *was very patient. She showed a lot of interest in her son's problem. She never blamed C or anyone else. She was willing to learn and understand. She understood that C was suffering and made it her goal to make things better for him. The seizures were under control. He was showing very small and slow improvements in his communication. His behavior was much improved. His schoolwork was showing gradual progress.*

The questions that arose in my mind in this case were the following: Were seizures a cause of autism in this child, or an association? Could there be other causes? Were the improvements shown due to the treatment of epilepsy or to other factors? What is the relationship between cognition, behavior and seizures?

Little C has verbal abilities, but what about people who don't? Many on the autism spectrum have no spoken language. Usually, these are more inclined to a seizure disorder. How can we decide with any confidence that these violent episodes and unusual behaviors are attention seeking or temper tantrums when they look like what is precisely described in the seizure literature? The relationships between epilepsy, language, behavior and cognition are not well understood. As far as Little C is concerned, seizures were clearly present and responded well to treatment.[70]

Testing the Theory of Seizures

Minshew asks the question, if a clinical presentation has the appearance of a certain disorder but the scientific corroboration is lacking –

---

70 Anand (2005).

as in a negative EEG – doesn't it makes sense to test the theory of the existence of seizure? Minshew believes it does.

It is logical too because it is well known that sometimes the tests do not show the seizures, so in those difficult cases, it becomes like trying to find a needle in a haystack. The key to understanding and deciphering each individual on the spectrum is akin to piecing together a puzzle after examining each piece carefully.

Since each person diagnosed with autism may have a different underlying pathology causing their particular autistic syndrome, we must take a closer look at each individual patient. We must look at the genes and inside the brain, and then ask the question, could partial epilepsy be a part of the scenario?

Only a physician can say for sure, but remember the signs to look for:

- Periods of blackout or confusion with memory impairment
- Occasional fainting spells with loss of bladder or bowel control followed by extreme fatigue
- Brief episodes of blank staring and brief periods where there is no response to questions
- Sudden falls for no apparent reason
- Episodes of blinking or chewing at inappropriate times
- A whole-body convulsion with or without a fever

If you notice any one or more of these, a discussion with a doctor is warranted.

CHAPTER 5

RECOGNIZING SILENT – OR PARTIAL – SEIZURES

Josh surveys the carnage of thrown objects and broken glass with profound confusion and sadness and then, while looking at his bloody hands, asks me, "Mom, what happened?"

Josh's silent seizures are sudden and unprovoked. They always begin with a vacant stare, and then it appears that he is having auditory (sound) and visual (seeing) hallucinations.

"I hate monsters with one eye," he roars. He then yells to the one-eyed monster, "Shut the hell up you mother f..."

He covers his ears. "I hear crunching potato chips in my ears and it's so loud," he cries out.

Sometimes at the very beginning of a seizure, he smiles for a brief moment in the midst of all the chaos. Often that smile is followed by a terrifying scream. His pupils dilate and a piercing scream fills the air. He clenches his teeth and proceeds to pull out a clump of his curly hair, soon thereafter opening his hand – slowly his blond locks waft towards the floor.

I hear that all-too-familiar scream, and without a thought I traverse the staircase, two stairs at a time. I try to speak with my son before he succumbs completely to this altered state. I want him to lie on his bed to minimize the potential for injury, so I try to guide him there while firmly speaking to him, "Get on your bed now!"

In the early stages of a seizure, he is able to listen and follow directions, but once it begins to spread across his brain, he cannot be reached. Quickly his behavior deteriorates into a form of internal madness. His body is reacting, too.

First I see his right foot moving. Then, in rapid succession, his face produces an unfamiliar contortion resembling a grimace and his eyelids flutter.

Suddenly, he punches the wall with his bare fists and says, "Ouch;" yet he continues. In a split second, he brings his fist to his mouth and bites down hard onto his hand, sinking his teeth deeply into his already scarred flesh, leaving deep red impressions, just as he did the last time, and the time before that.

His breathing gradually returns to normal. He is in obvious pain as he stares at his hand, trying to understand all that has just occurred.

As always, when it is over, he is perplexed and remorseful. It is obvious that he cannot control these visions of one-eyed monsters that accompany his seizure or the distorted sounds they hurl at his sensitive ears. He has some awareness that he is responsible for the carnage, and in calmer moments he taps his head and says, "I need to control your head." [Like so many with autism, Josh sometimes reverses his pronouns and uses "your" instead of "my."]

Imagine experiencing this kind of horror and the physical pain, being unable to properly express what you are experiencing, and feeling that somehow you are responsible for it and must learn to control it.

In the Absence of Visible Signs

An "absence seizure" (formerly called *petit mal seizure*) produces a sudden loss of consciousness in a person with epilepsy. The person appears to "blank out" and may not remember the brief episode later.

I had an opportunity to witness this type of seizure first-hand years ago. My college roommate's sister had epilepsy, and numerous times a day she would stare into space blankly for periods of 15 to 30 seconds. At the time, I found it strange and interesting as she simply "zoned out" and then, blinking her eyes, suddenly came back. I would have assumed she was daydreaming, but she shared her medical history with me, so I knew what was happening.

My memory of that experience came back when Josh began his episodes of staring at nothing, at nobody, into some unreachable alternate universe beyond my reach and immune to my love. I recalled seeing my roommate's sister do the same thing ... she would simply stop and stare into space at nothing. Although she was deemed normal in every way, she was visited multiple times a day by these "silent seizures."

In the preface of her book *Seized*, author Eve LaPlante says that this kinds of seizure, also called temporal lobe epilepsy, affects one million Americans, and she estimates another million go undiagnosed.[71] When most people think of seizures, they think of the variety that cause a person to collapse into tonic-clonic convulsions (see Chapter 4), which involve violent muscle spasms and loss of

---

71 LaPlante (1993, 2000).

consciousness. Most of us are not familiar with the *partial* type of seizure that can go undetected and, therefore, is easily missed. But today, some specialists in the area of autism spectrum disorders are beginning to realize that subclinical seizures play a big role in this perplexing disorder.[72]

Recognizing these silent seizures, particularly the simple and complex partial variety (see Chapter 4), requires the ability to objectively detect subtle changes in the person's behavior and subsequent deterioration of his or her abilities. This is a difficult challenge, requiring intimate knowledge about the person's level of general functioning. Most physicians don't have such knowledge and, therefore, must rely mainly on the reports and observations of caregivers. And this is why it is so important that our observations and subsequent reports are as comprehensive, detailed and accurate as possible (see Chapter 6).

As parents, we know best how our children function when they are not seizing. Medical professionals are naturally less in tune with the child's everyday "normal" behavior and understandably can mistake unusual behaviors as mere manifestations of intellectual disability or some behavioral manifestation.

"Tragically, there is a pervasive reluctance to make a clinical diagnosis of seizure when scientific EEG corroboration is lacking," states Dr. Minshew. "Making the diagnosis of partial epilepsy seems to be a catch-22. If a person is just acting strangely, there are many explanations other than seizure, and yet if a person falls to the ground while her whole body is shaking, there isn't another diagnosis that would make sense. We all have preconceived notions that we hold on to, but we must learn to let go of these if we are to care well for these patients."[73]

---

72 N. Minshew (personal communication, June 4, 2008).
73 N. Minshew (personal communication, June 4, 2008).

Minshew notes that in medical practice, too much emphasis is placed upon the abnormal EEG findings. Josh has never had an abnormal EEG according to those who interpret them. Yet, he exhibits all of the signs and symptoms of a partial seizure disorder. Dr. Taff was convinced seizures exist *solely* based upon the absence of language and the compelling staring spells.

If I had decided to take the negative EEG at face value, the consequences would have been devastating. Caregivers, teachers and physicians may have an intellectual awareness of the characteristics of a partial seizure, yet may never have seen one occur.

Signs of a Partial Seizure

Minshew explains that a seizure profile consists of the following three distinct phases. Being able to identify these stages will facilitate coping with what can be a highly stressful circumstance and help parents and other caregivers minimize any potential harm to the child:

1. The person is behaving at a typical level of functioning. (Understanding the child's normal way of behaving.)

2. The seizure erupts without warning or provocation, disrupting the normal functioning of the seizing person and producing very different behavior from what was displayed just moments before.

3. An abrupt return follows from the seizure state back to the normal state as the seizure comes to an end.

Minshew highlights the importance of noting this *episodic* change in the behavior. If the behavior is brief and seems mild, it may easily go unrecognized as an ictal (seizure; see Chapter 4) event, since consciousness was only momentarily altered and /or lost.

A seizure can present at various times in life, including the three critical periods in the life of a child:

1. Prior to the age of 2

2. 6-8 years of age, the first "brain pruning period"[74]

3. Puberty

The casual observer without any understanding of partial epilepsy could easily surmise that a person who is staring and momentarily "zoning out" is merely lost in thought or daydreaming. As time passes and the episodes become more frequent and more severe, the clinician can feel more confident about making the diagnosis of a seizure disorder.

A number of visual signs can indicate the onset of a seizure. These signs follow a pattern that is much the same in every episode, as described below.

Signs That Can Signal the Onset of a Seizure

- Sudden changes in behavior with complete halting of the previous activity, such as a sudden eruption of fear that may manifest as screaming or the person seeming to be in a trance, and not capable of responding normally. The person may complain of seeing a vision or having a visual problem, such as seeing black dots or a temporary loss of all or partial vision.

- Enlarging pupils: The center portion of the eye or pupil becomes much larger than normal, and the eyes may gaze to one side.

- Staring: Fixed stare and loss of awareness of surroundings, which looks like daydreaming or a trance-like state. The individual will seem as if he is sleepwalking.

---

74 *Seizures.* http://www.tacanow.org/family-resources/seizures/

- Inability to understand language: The person may not respond in a manner that is "normal" for him when asked, "Are you OK?" or may respond inappropriately.

- Possible clicking sounds with the tongue.

- Changes in the ability to communicate, such as seeming incoherent and saying things that make no sense, called gibberish. This could be an attempt to describe to you what is occurring. Josh says, "The man put duct tape on my mouth and tried to hurt me" or "Sammy is bothering me."

- Temper tantrums or aggression: Screaming, hair pulling, fighting, kicking, biting or what seems like a random flailing or an attempt to fight off an intruder. This is directed to whomever is nearest, or to themselves.

- Self-injury, including head-banging, biting, punching self and slapping head.

- Eye blinking, staring, facial grimacing, odd movements, lip biting and chewing.

- Seeing things that are not there (visual hallucinations). These may include Ninjas, God, incredibly beautiful scenes, one-eyed monsters or gargoyles.

- Hearing things that are not there (auditory hallucinations).

- Sensory hallucinations: Smelling something not there, such as a burning smell; odd feelings described as funny sensations in the stomach.

- Hypergraphia: Some people describe an intense need to write compulsively.

- Hyper-religiosity: A very intense interest in religion and God.[75]

---

75 N. Minshew (personal communication, June 4, 2008).

After a seizure, there is often a period of confusion lasting minutes, possibly followed by a sudden attack of sleepiness and fatigue. Beware of this, especially if the child has outgrown napping.

Tips for How to Prevent and Address Seizures

- Give medications consistently and query your child's doctor if frequent prescription changes are made. Medication changes can precipitate a seizure, and some medications lower the seizure threshold, making it more likely that a seizure will occur.

- Avoid missing a scheduled dose of medication; this is risking a seizure.

- Maintain a therapeutic dose of any medication; this is crucial to ensure the medication is targeting the problem.

- Ensure that the child gets plenty of sleep with a regular bed time and adequate rest periods during the day. Lack of sleep can worsen a seizure disorder. Seizures are often observed when a child wakes in the morning and/or later in the day when fatigue sets in.

- Be aware that illness can lower the seizure threshold, making a seizure more likely to occur, especially during the incubation period when the child is "coming down with something."

- Avoid flickering lights such as strobes, as they can induce seizure.

- Monitor blood sugar levels: Both low and high blood sugar levels can cause a seizure.

- Help the child avoid stress; stress lowers the threshold of seizure.

- Parents of teenagers, be aware that alcohol can lower the seizure threshold and counsel children accordingly.

- Make sure the child eats regular meals consisting of healthy foods; this is very important for optimal brain function.

- Stick to a low sugar diet.

- Avoid aspartame (Nutrasweet). In my experience, it lowers the seizure threshold, and Josh's doctor has removed it from is diet.

Diagnosing silent seizures depends on being able to recognize the recurrent pattern in the deterioration of the level of functioning and noticing the odd behavior, which is abrupt in its onset and quite brief. **It can be as brief as a 5- to 30-second staring spell and a fleeting facial grimace with eye flutter.**

It can be an overwhelming challenge for the person living with these silent seizures. Many are confronted by anger and falsely accused of disorderly conduct, indecent exposure and drug abuse – some are even unfairly arrested. Bizarre actions exhibited during a seizure have led to frequent misdiagnosis, medical mismanagement, expulsion from school and, in the worst case, commitment to a mental institution.

We must help our loved ones be understood. We have to give a voice to their suffering. Trust your instincts as parents. Never give up on helping your child to be the best that he or she can be. Parents need to be partners with their child's doctors, and together unravel this puzzle known as autism.

CHAPTER 6

DIAGNOSING AND TREATING SEIZURES AND CO-OCCURRING CONDITIONS

I recommend that, whenever possible, parents who suspect their child may have a silent seizure disorder consult with a team of physicians who specialize in autism rather than taking the word of one doctor. The team should, preferably, include a professor of neurology and psychiatry with expertise in the cognitive issues found in autism and a behavioral specialist who can dissect the troubling behaviors to determine whether there is any external provocation or not. For example, if a person with autism is upset because he is not getting something he wants, that would be important to note versus an episodic rage attack that has no discernible cause. The remedy for each issue is entirely different. The random rage attack from either the seizure or the psychosis would be treated with medication, whereas a tantrum in response to frustration would require the employment of behavioral techniques.

Behavioral data sheets and other logs are useful tools in the attempt to dissect and understand a given behavior, which in turn helps the physician to understand what treatment is needed (see samples on pp. 90-95).

Parents should also ask for the most up-to-date, comprehensive genetic testing to assess all possible underlying causes of autistic behaviors. Genetic and environmental factors also influence development, so a thorough prenatal history and maternal exposures should be discussed.

A specific diagnosis, if one is found, will provide families with a clearer understanding of the nature of the disorder, the expected outcome and the risks involved in future pregnancies. Knowledge is power, particularly when it comes to disease states. Leave no stone unturned. Some of the tests that may be useful in yielding a diagnosis are listed below.[76]

Medical Tests to Identify Underlying Causes of Autism That May Influence the Ultimate Prognosis
• DNA microarray test for all known genetic disorders linked to autism, specifically high-resolution chromosome analysis • PKU • Audiological examination • Thyroid function • Lipid profiles, including long-chain fatty acids • Blood chemistry and CBC (complete blood count) panel • Micronutrients, such as vitamin levels (including vitamins E, B-12, D, and folate) • Ammonia level • Celiac antibodies • Carnitine (involved in fatty acid metabolism) • Toxoplasma IgG (toxoplasmosis is a serious illness that occurs when a fetus is infected with the parasite that causes this disease). Some affected newborns have brain damage as a result. This test, if positive, will detect the antibodies and lead to a diagnosis.

76 Aetna (n.d.).

Medical Tests to Identify Underlying Causes of Autism That May Influence the Ultimate Prognosis (cont.)

- Hepatic function (liver)
- Heavy metal and lead screening
- Pyruvate and arterial lactic acid levels
- Amino and organic acid screening
- Cytomegalovirus screening
- Urinary peptides
- Noninvasive imaging, including:
  - EEG, in particular dense-array EEG: Dense-array EEG is an improvement on the standard because it uses a larger number of electrodes so there is improved accuracy. This method is particularly useful in detecting subclinical seizures.
  - Sleep-deprived EEG if there is a high suspicion of subclinical seizures or symptoms of regression
  - Video EEG
  - MRI (magnetic resonance imaging)
  - MRS (magnetic resonance spectroscopy)
  - PET (positron emission tomography)
  - MEG (magentoencephalography)
  - Allergy testing for environmental causes such as mold
  - Allergy testing for foods such as gluten and casein

The above tests are not ordered routinely by physicians. Therefore, it is incumbent upon the family to request them. If encountering resistance, don't take no for an answer. It is too important. (The cost may be covered by insurance or the Medicaid waiver, when appropriate.) Many of the tests listed above were ordered for Josh by his team of physicians, which is how I became familiar with them. In addition, from my insurance carrier, I obtained a list of approved and covered tests that aid in arriving at a definitive diagnosis (see footnote #76).

Understanding Your Child's Behavior

All behavior has a purpose. Therefore, even the most "unusual" manifestations warrant careful attention as part of the process of getting an accurate picture of the child's autism. Parents are often told that many of the problematic behaviors they report are just "a part of autism," when in fact we have learned that many of them can be signs of partial seizures. A patient having a partial seizure can experience a range of strange and unusual sensations, jerking of a body part, distortion of vision or sound, hallucinations or a sudden sense of fear. These seizures alter perception and negatively impact behavior.

Imagine for one moment having a partial seizure disorder that conjures up hallucinations, delusions and frightening visions from the past. On top of that, you may have little or no ability to communicate what is happening to you. You might feel frightened and anxious, and because you lack adequate language ability, you resort to behaviors to express what is happening. You might scream, hold your ears to keep the voices quiet, or throw an aggressive tantrum to thwart the attack you are experiencing. Confusion, panic and fear escalate as you desperately try to be understood.

The fact that this seizure "component of autism" can be discovered by astute observation, and subsequently treated, continues to be overlooked by the professionals we seek out when our children are initially diagnosed. It is important to remember this key point: *When seizures continue unabated, they wreak havoc on a developing brain.* Therefore, it is critical that they be recognized and treated as early as possible.

However, even for someone diagnosed with autism as long as 15 or 20 years ago, treating the seizure component now can have a dramatic effect on overall functioning. The diagnosis of autism, regardless of the origins, has many treatable facets, so it's worthwhile to pursue a more comprehensive diagnosis of all the facets involved. My personal experience suggests that when it comes to accurate diagnosis of the underlying conditions associated with autism, earlier – *before extensive damage is done* – is far better than later. However, it is never too late to unlock a child's potential. At age 24, my son is in community college (with a peer assistant) pursuing his dream of attending school at his functioning level. He is non-matriculated, but he is finally blending in as "one of the guys."

Analyzing the behavior is an essential first step in accurate diagnosis. Usually a behavioral specialist can assist in this regard. (Behavioral specialists hold credentials with these identifying letters, BCBA: behavioral consultant, behavioral analyst.) You may request a consultation through your school district, especially if the behavior occurs at school. Another option is to inquire if a consult is covered by your insurance and then hiring a consultant yourself. Be sure to look for a highly trained, experienced person to conduct the assessment.

A functional behavioral assessment (FBA), which is a study and analysis of behavior in a given person, should be requested when a student presents with challenging behavior such as aggression and/or the presentation of symptoms of partial seizures. The FBA looks beyond the behavior itself, and attempts to understand if environmental, social and medical factors might be contributing. The psychologist or behavior analyst conducting the FBA observes the student in different settings and conducts interviews with as many people as possible in the person's life, such as teachers, staff and parents.

The functional analysis should attempt to answer the following questions:

- What is the problem behavior?

- At what time of day has it occurred? Is there a pattern to this time of day?

- Frequency, time elapsed and grade: mild, moderate or severe?

- Was the person asking or seeming in need of something or was the behavior seemingly completely random?

- Were there flashing lights, loud sounds and a lot of stimulation?

- Who was present?

- What happened just prior to the behavior?

- What happened during and after?

- Did the person just take his medication or mistakenly skip a dose – that is, time relationship between last medication and "incident?"

Keep a daily log (see sample at the end of this chapter) of behavioral outbursts, the events surrounding and preceding them, as well as details regarding how much time lapsed. This kind of information will assist in understanding the origin of the troubling behavior. If the behavior is deemed to have no function to the person, this might indicate that a silent seizure disorder is the culprit.

Suspecting a seizure disorder is the first step in a multi-step process. If you think your child might be silently seizing, call a neurologist or psychiatrist who has expertise in autism. If you encounter resistance to a suggestion of subclinical seizures, do not let that deter you, as repeated throughout this book. Many medical centers have teams who specialize in autism such as the team we use at Columbia Medical Center. (Check with a major organization such as Autism Speaks for more information on options.)

Prepare for the initial consultation with your chosen physician by bringing all the essential information gathered by the FBA and your own diary log of events. To get an accurate diagnosis, a physician will want a thorough history of the patient, in as much depth as possible, starting from birth.

It will be important for the treating physician to ascertain whether a seizure disorder is present and whether the symptoms may be ascribed to a particular syndrome in which seizure and autism might co-exist. As we have discussed, many genetic syndromes have similar symptoms, yet very different underlying problems. Many of these syndromes can be detected now through blood testing.

After the initial visit, the next step is usually a clinical evaluation, which should include brain testing to search for the underlying cause. The doctor's main tools for determining the cause, in addition to dense-array EEG (see p. 80) and MRI, are a thorough medical history and a detailed understanding of what is occurring now, based on caregiver observations. That is why it is essential to keep a diary with all the pertinent information.

Ultimately, collecting the relevant data will help guide the treatment plan. Thus, it is critical that the data be as accurate as possible. Many seizure types have similar symptoms but with subtle differences. Describing all symptoms to the physician will help him or her choose the right treatment, including medication.

Helpful Data for Parents to Collect for the Neurologist Looking to See if a Silent Seizure Disorder Is Present:

Was the patient ...

- Aware that a seizure was starting?

- Aware of any aura?[77]

---

77 An aura is a distinctive feeling or some other warning sign that indicates a seizure is coming on.

- Appearing to be seeing or hearing things at the onset or during the seizure?

- Doing anything prior, such as watching TV or looking at a strobe light?

- Exhibiting any staring, lip smacking, facial grimacing, eye fluttering or screaming?

- Able to respond at any point?

- Exhibiting stiffening of the body or movement in the limbs? If so, which side of the body?

- Clenching jaw or biting down hard on an object or him/herself?

- Incontinent of urine or feces?

- Aggressive or violent at any point during the seizure and, if so, was the behavior directed at anyone?

- Complaining of head pain either before or after the seizure?

- Sleepy afterward and, if so, for how long?

Remember ...

The diagnosis of subclinical silent seizures in individuals with intellectual impairments is primarily a *clinical* one, which means it is based on physical observation, accurate descriptions and a detailed history, as opposed to concrete evidence via the results of an EEG or MRI. Many doctors rely on a thorough, detailed description of the entire episode. If the patient cannot communicate about the episode, the physician must rely on eyewitness accounts. Videotaping episodes can be helpful, although *visually*, these spells are often misleading and *look like* psychotic episodes.

If the child can draw what is happening, that can sometimes be helpful. Josh drew three people inside his head and a fourth on the outside yelling in his ear. He also drew a boy in a bed with his eyes twitching and wrote in a cartoon bubble,"It has a funny smell."This was immensely helpful. Hallucinated smells, especially "burning," are classic symptoms of temporal lope epilepsy!

Dr. Minshew explains:

Routine EEGs sometimes detect the abnormal electrical patterns in the brain, which is helpful in categorizing and localizing many seizure types. EEGs are only helpful when they are confirming the diagnosis of a seizure. If it is positive at the time the problem behavior is occurring, it is easier to make the diagnosis of seizure. Since the EEG can only monitor the top portion of the brain's cortex, a vast area is left completely unexplored. As neurologists know, frontal and temporal lobes are very potent generators of seizures, and tragically for these patients [whose seizures are in those areas], this method often fails to detect them.[78]

Science Behind the Theory: The Ah-ha! Moment

Dr. Minshew tells a story about a group of patients who had exhibited bizarre behaviors and were labeled "hysterics" by their doctors after having routine surface EEGs (via electrodes applied only to the scalp) that registered "negative" for seizure. The doctors felt there might be more to the story and pursued a more in-depth test in an effort to prove their suspicion of seizure. The patients subsequently underwent implantation of depth electrodes inside their skulls (a test called *transphenoidal EEG,* in which electrodes are inserted through the nostrils while the patient is sedated). This test has been used successfully to prove seizures that exist in a given patient, though it is poorly tol-

---

78 N. Minshew (personal communication, June 4, 2008).

erated. The results of this test were very illuminating. Much to the surprise of the doctors, this EEG registered spikes indicating a seizure disorder, which correlated to bouts of odd behavior. As a result, their diagnosis changed from "hysterics" to "seizure."

It's important to note that routine surface EEGs in all these patients were read as negative for seizure, or normal. The depth electrodes implanted in their skulls finally showed the electrical discharges, but the test required a surgical procedure that is invasive and poorly tolerated by most patients and, therefore, is seldom done any more. Based on such experiences, Dr. Minshew reminds us to be vigilant and open-minded in the face of science, which is inexact and always evolving.

The EEG Bottom Line

An EEG should be performed in all suspected cases of seizure, with the understanding that the resultant information is limited in the overall diagnosis of epilepsy. Newer technologies may be helpful in discovering abnormal electrical discharges in the brain; for example, dense-array EEGs use a much larger number of electrodes, resulting in better accuracy and localization of any electrical discharges.

Dr. Fernando Miranda, a San Francisco, California, neurologist who treats children on the autism spectrum and understands the co-existence of seizures in autism, shares the following information related to the autism-seizure connection.

The disorder commonly referred to as autism is currently diagnosed almost entirely on the basis of observable behavioral symptoms, which clearly is not optimal. An analysis of the brain is needed for proper diagnosis, and is an essential com-

ponent which is often overlooked. Additionally, the means of analyzing the information must also be effective if we, as doctors, are going to make accurate conclusions.

Two statements about autism are unequivocal. First, autism is a disorder that is localized in the central nervous system, more specifically inside the brain. Second, the behavior markers that lead a physician to suspect autism – such as language impairments, stereotyped behavior, impaired social interaction and, for some, associated intellectual disability – do not provide a clear indication of where in the brain the problems arise.

Thus, at this point in time, it is safe to say that autism being diagnosed only on the basis of observed behavioral symptoms without looking inside the brain is analogous to an ophthalmologist observing blurry vision in a person who complains of reading difficulty, conducting no in-depth eye exam and telling the patient she is near-sighted. Who in their right mind would trust such a minimal assessment? Many of us do …

In the practice of neurology, all behavioral observations should be augmented with objective and quantifiable testing that examines the brain in much the same way an eye doctor examines the eyes. The doctor uses all the appropriate tools at his or her disposal before making any solid diagnosis or prescribing any kind of treatment.

The importance of using MRI as a tool in diagnosis is well established. We use MRI to look at the anatomy of the brain, specifically to look for any abnormalities. (MRI SPECT scanning is then used to study the composition of the brain.) MRI SPECT scanning can indicate the presence or absence of cell abnormalities in the white matter of the brain.

In addition to examining the structure and chemical composition, it is crucial to examine brain function. The language hemisphere of the brain is quite complex. Columns of nerve cells each perform a specific function. In children with autism, these columns of nerve cells become disarranged either due to injury or destruction of the nerve fibers, leading to interruption or elimination of nerve impulses. This process is called "de-affernation."

When nerves do not receive the appropriate enervation, they become hyperactive. When this happens, there is a clinical manifestation, which causes a sudden electrical discharge from the brain.

Using a more advanced dense-array EEG, in my practice of neurology, we have been successfully identifying such paroxysmal (sudden) discharges in 60-70 percent of children with ASD. Moreover, a conservative estimate is that up to 40 percent of children diagnosed with ASD will have, or have had, at least one or two generalized seizures in their lifetime. This is a larger number than we had previously thought.

It is extremely important to identify the presence or absence of paroxysmal discharges in children diagnosed with ASD and then to determine the right antiseizure medication to control them. Many of the antiseizure medications currently available, such as Lamictal, produce very little, if any, cognitive side effects.

It is also crucial to obtain a sleep EEG, since the majority (80 percent) of seizure discharges occur either during sleep or in the transition between sleep and wakefulness. Neuropsychological testing is beneficial as well, so that doctors can pinpoint each child's unique areas of strength. We want to keep learning how to best apply diagnostic tools. Freedom from seizures *is the goal! Neurologists should be more involved in the fight to better understand and treat autism spectrum disorders which we are certain begin in the brain.*

Pitfalls in the Current Testing Model

EEG testing has limitations. Specifically, it may be negative in some cases of partial seizures, especially when the discharge originates in the frontal lobe of the brain.[79]

To look deeper into the suspected seizure activity, Dr. Miranda suggest, video monitoring is helpful, and is best done when a patient is admitted to the hospital and has a continuous EEG for a defined period of time – usually three to five days. As an option, patients can undergo an ambulatory EEG, which uses a small portable machine with leads attached to the scalp and worn as a shoulder bag. Any seizures that occur during the testing period are recorded by either method, *as long as they occur in an area of the brain where the electrodes can detect them.* A newer technology, called dense-array EEG, tends to be better at picking up the erratic electrical impulses and is being used by Dr. Miranda with success.[80]

Medication Used to Treat Seizures

The following is Dr. Miranda's views and experiences with use of medication.

The majority of seizures can be controlled by medications. If there is a high suspicion that a person has a subclinical seizure

---

79 Favors (2009).
80 F. Miranda (personal communication, June 4, 2008).

disorder, it is important to consider daily medication control. Medications are considered the first line of treatment (best first option available) for seizure control.

Seizure medications are making a huge difference for children with subclinical seizures. We must thoroughly assess all children who receive this diagnosis of ASD and look inside their brain in depth to determine what exactly is going on. These seizures are often invisible to the naked eye, but they continue to cause injury to the developing brain and, if allowed to continue, often lead to deleterious effects.

There is no harm in trying a patient on a course of antiseizure medication to see if behavior and cognition improve. In my practice, we are seeing incredible successes treating patients with ASD with medication aimed at seizure control. Many of these children are becoming included in general education classrooms at school as they begin to speak and learn. We are happy to report that many of them are becoming indistinguishable from their typical peers.

Choice of medication should be made after very careful consideration and counsel, preferably with a team of medical doctors comprised of a neurologist, a psychiatrist, and a behavioral psychologist, all of whom ideally understand the connection between epilepsy and autism. The choice of medication will depend on the seizure type, and should include consideration of any co-existing conditions as well as any medications the patient is already taking. This is especially important because some medications given for co-occurring conditions can lower a resistance to seizures, making a seizure more likely to occur. Other factors to consider when choosing a medication include *safety and side effects. It is important to discuss with the pre-scribing physician the best way to achieve a constant level of medication in the blood. Some preparations have an extended release, which helps to achieve a constant blood level.*

Medications are typically administered in trial periods, dur-ing which the patient/family and doctor assess the benefits vs. risks. The medication's effectiveness should be evaluated when it reaches the therapeutic level, which is medication-specific (a therapeutic level is the level at which a medication is at a dose high enough to produce the desired effect). Every effort should be made to attain seizure control, but even a reduction in the num-ber of seizures is a positive step.

Important: Severe psychotic behavioral changes can result when seizures are being controlled, a process called "forced normalization." The psychosis can be acute (comes and goes) or chronic (stays constant). The psychosis requires treatment and must be recognized as such. An antipsychotic, such as Risperadol, is often prescribed together with the antiseizure medication.

Risperadol has been a good choice for Josh. At a ther-apeutic dose of 4 mg, his psychotic ninja-kicking epi-sodes are completely controlled. Though 4 mg works for Josh, each patient needs an individualized dose to be determined with counsel from a psychiatrist or neu-rologist. Often the person's body weight is an impor-tant factor in determining the amount of a medication to be prescribed.

Patients taking these preparations may experience side effects. They may be mild and dissipate over time, or they may prove in-tolerable. Discuss medications and the possible side effects with your child's physician prior to starting any new medication.[81]

Monitoring

"Low and slow" applies to beginning any new medication. Small, incremental changes are the way to go, whether increasing or decreasing a medication. Take the time to assess how it is working and then slowly adjust. When it comes to adding or subtracting medications, *only make one change at a time* so you can accurately identify the effects of each one. This is very important.

Some medications, such as Depakote, require that blood levels be checked periodically so as to maintain a safe amount of drug in the body. There is a time of day when a medicine "peaks" (highest level) and when it "troughs" (lowest level), which can be different for every medication.

For most individuals on anticonvulsant regimens, the trough occurs in the morning prior to the patient's first dose. This is the best time to take a blood sample to test for the level of medication in the blood. This information should be the doctor's responsibility to know and share with you.

Even if a blood level is higher than the standard reference range, it might be okay to stay on the medication as long as it is not causing any adverse side effects. Always discuss the situation in depth with your doctor. Sometimes people do just great with slightly higher levels of medicine, and since it might make a big difference, it should be pursued.

---

81 F. Miranda (personal communication, June 4, 2008).

> Generic medications are fine except when it comes to seizure medications. Josh did very poorly on generic preparations. Beware of them!

Treating all of the co-occurring conditions is the best way to achieve overall wellness and remediation of symptoms.

1. The partial seizure in Josh produces odd behaviors and aggression, including brief staring spells, followed by odd verbal gibberish, facial grimacing, hair pulling, clenching teeth and biting. The antiseizure medicine Depakote DR (delayed release) has helped to suppress these seizures. Josh's physician felt that maintaining a therapeutic range based upon his weight would provide a cessation of the seizures. The Depakote seems to work very well for his overall seizure control.

2. Josh's psychotic symptoms are aggressive or combat-like in nature as he tries to fend off the ninja attacks. Whether the psychosis is produced within the seizure, between seizures, or as a separate entity is almost impossible to discern. It has been successfully treated with Risperadol, which must be given at a therapeutic level, meaning enough of the medicine to quell a psychosis.

> "Oculogyric crisis" is a side effect of neuroleptic medication such as Risperadol; it causes the eyes to move at random, either up, down, or side-to-side. Additionally, irritability and aggression can be seen. Josh's doctor prescribed a medication used to the treat side effects called Cogentin, which has helped him immeasurably.

3. Depression is common in individuals with seizures and ASD; Josh is being treated with Zoloft. It works very well for him.

4. Sleep problems is another common complaint. Josh suffered for years until he was prescribed Trazedone. He sleeps very well now.

What to Do When a Seizure Begins

Seizures can be very scary to witness and cause anxiety in the observer, but it is important to try to stay calm. Astute observation and common sense are helpful. In addition, here is a list of best practices.

1. Get the person to a safe place, away from sharp objects, such as bed or sofa with pillows placed around the person. (It is best for the person not to wander, since she is unaware of her surroundings and at risk for behavior that could produce a hazard if near fire or a stove, climbing heights or operating machinery.)

2. Provide emotional support. Speak in a calm, reassuring manner. "You are having a seizure, but it will pass. I am here to help you."

3. If a violent seizure happens in public, try to reassure the startled people around you to deflect the attention such a seizure will almost inevitably bring. In my personal experience, I noted that if others realize what is occurring, they become more at ease and seem to show more compassion and understanding.

4. Remember that seizures can be deadly. If you suspect your child has seizures, seek medical help to guide you toward proper treatment. Sometimes, even with treatment, accidents occur. But the likelihood of severe consequences increases in the absence of treatment.

The tragic story of John Travolta's son Jett, suspected to have autism and confirmed to have seizures, should be a wake-up call to all of us. It demonstrates what can happen as a result of a seizure disorder when medication is withdrawn. According to a *People* magazine interview after his son's death, John Travolta told a court that "every 5 to 10 days Jett would have seizures lasting 45 seconds to one minute, and then he would sleep for 12 hours." Seizure disorders are among the leading causes of death in people with autism, according to a study cited in the article.[82]

A condition known as SUDEP (Sudden Death in Epilepsy) is characterized by sudden death with no discernible cause identified. Individuals with intellectual disabilities are vulnerable to this, especially when there is a pattern of erratic medication administration or a history of taking sub-therapeutic doses of anticonvulsants (that is, the medication dose is too low and, therefore, ineffective at seizure control).[83]

Times When Emergency Help Is Appropriate

- If a seizure happens in water

- If there is no way to learn if the seizure is caused by epilepsy

- If the person is injured, pregnant or diabetic

- If the seizure continues – for longer than 5 minutes

- If a second seizure starts shortly after the first has ended

- If consciousness does not return after the convulsions have stopped

Knowledge is power. Make it a practice to empower yourself and others. None of us chose this club we find ourselves in, yet here we are. We can learn from each other's mistakes and triumphs, and in doing so help countless other families.

---

82 Marikar, Childs, & Chitale (2009).
83 N. Minshew (personal communication, June 4, 2008).

Sample Medication Log

DATE	TIME	MEDICATION	DOSE

Sample Behavior Data Sheet

Make a copy of this form and fill it out following *all* instances of aggression, screaming, self-injury or other problem behaviors.

Date:
Time:
Duration:
Location:
Persons Present:
Time of Last Medication:
Last Medication Given + Dose:
Behavior: (Be specific. Instead of saying "outburst" describe the specific behavior: "screaming,""yelling,""stomping,""banging head on the floor," etc.)
Antecedent: (What happened immediately before the behavior? Include what the person was doing, what others were doing, and any precursor behaviors such as eye movements, foot tapping, etc.)

Book Diary

Date:_____Time:_____Length:____min. ____sec.	☐　**Flag It**

Type:　☐ Simple Partial　☐ Complex Partial　☐ Secondary Generalized　☐ Atonic
☐ Tonic　☐ Clonic　☐ Tonic-Clonic　☐ Myoclonic　☐ Atypical Absence
☐ Absence　☐ Infantile Spasms (cluster)　☐ Unknown

Mood:　☐ Good ☐ Normal ☐ Bad	**OTC Medications**_____

Possible Triggers:　　　☐ Changes in Medication (including late or missed)

☐ Overtired or irregular sleep　☐ Alcohol or drug use　☐ Irregular Diet

☐ Bright or flashing lights　☐ Fever or overheated　☐ Emotional Stress

☐ Hormonal fluctuations　☐ Sick – *Describe*_____

☐ Other_____

Trigger notes: _____

_____

_____

Description:　　☐ Change in awareness ☐ Loss of urine or bowel control

☐ Loss of ability to communicate　　　☐ Automatic repeated movements

☐ Muscle stiffness in_____　　　☐ Aura

☐ Muscle twitch in_____　　　☐ Other_____

Description notes: _____

_____

_____

Post event:　　☐ Unable to communicate　☐ Remembers event

☐ Sleepy　　　☐ Muscle weakness　　　☐ Sleepy

Post event notes: _____

_____

_____

Date:_____**Time**:_____**Length**:____min. ____sec.	☐ **Flag It**

Type: ☐ Simple Partial ☐ Complex Partial ☐ Secondary Generalized ☐ Atonic
☐ Tonic ☐ Clonic ☐ Tonic-Clonic ☐ Myoclonic ☐ Atypical Absence
☐ Absence ☐ Infantile Spasms (cluster) ☐ Unknown

Mood: ☐ Good ☐ Normal ☐ Bad	**OTC Medications**_____

Possible Triggers: ☐ Changes in Medication (including late or missed)

☐ Overtired or irregular sleep ☐ Alcohol or drug use ☐ Irregular Diet

☐ Bright or flashing lights ☐ Fever or overheated ☐ Emotional Stress

☐ Hormonal fluctuations ☐ Sick – *Describe*_____

☐ Other_____

Trigger notes: _____
_____
_____

Description: ☐ Change in awareness ☐ Loss of urine or bowel control

☐ Loss of ability to communicate ☐ Automatic repeated movements

☐ Muscle stiffness in_____ ☐ Aura

☐ Muscle twitch in_____ ☐ Other_____

Description notes: _____
_____
_____
_____

Post event: ☐ Unable to communicate ☐ Remembers event

☐ Sleepy ☐ Muscle weakness ☐ Sleepy

Post event notes: _____
_____
_____

| Date:_____ Time:_____ Length:____min. ____sec. | ☐ **Flag It** |

Type: ☐ Simple Partial ☐ Complex Partial ☐ Secondary Generalized ☐ Atonic
☐ Tonic ☐ Clonic ☐ Tonic-Clonic ☐ Myoclonic ☐ Atypical Absence
☐ Absence ☐ Infantile Spasms (cluster) ☐ Unknown

Mood: ☐ Good ☐ Normal ☐ Bad | **OTC Medications**_____

Possible Triggers: ☐ Changes in Medication (including late or missed)

☐ Overtired or irregular sleep ☐ Alcohol or drug use ☐ Irregular Diet

☐ Bright or flashing lights ☐ Fever or overheated ☐ Emotional Stress

☐ Hormonal fluctuations ☐ Sick – *Describe*_____

☐ Other_____

Trigger notes: _____
_____
_____

Description: ☐ Change in awareness ☐ Loss of urine or bowel control

☐ Loss of ability to communicate   ☐ Automatic repeated movements

☐ Muscle stiffness in_____   ☐ Aura

☐ Muscle twitch in_____   ☐ Other_____

Description notes: _____
_____
_____
_____

Post event: ☐ Unable to communicate ☐ Remembers event

☐ Sleepy   ☐ Muscle weakness   ☐ Sleepy

Post event notes: _____
_____
_____

Date:_____ Time:_____ Length:____min. ____sec.	☐ **Flag It**

Type: ☐ Simple Partial ☐ Complex Partial ☐ Secondary Generalized ☐ Atonic
☐ Tonic ☐ Clonic ☐ Tonic-Clonic ☐ Myoclonic ☐ Atypical Absence
☐ Absence ☐ Infantile Spasms (cluster) ☐ Unknown

Mood: ☐ Good ☐ Normal ☐ Bad	**OTC Medications**_____

Possible Triggers: ☐ Changes in Medication (including late or missed)

☐ Overtired or irregular sleep ☐ Alcohol or drug use ☐ Irregular Diet

☐ Bright or flashing lights ☐ Fever or overheated ☐ Emotional Stress

☐ Hormonal fluctuations ☐ Sick – *Describe*_____

☐ Other_____

Trigger notes: _____

_____

_____

Description: ☐ Change in awareness ☐ Loss of urine or bowel control

☐ Loss of ability to communicate   ☐ Automatic repeated movements

☐ Muscle stiffness in_____   ☐ Aura

☐ Muscle twitch in_____   ☐ Other_____

Description notes: _____

_____

_____

_____

Post event: ☐ Unable to communicate ☐ Remembers event

☐ Sleepy   ☐ Muscle weakness   ☐ Sleepy

Post event notes: _____

_____

_____

This form and more are downloadable at www.SeizureTracker.com/MainSuppDocs.php.

CHAPTER 7

NEUROFEEDBACK AND OTHER PROMISING TREATMENTS

Τhis chapter presents the results of current research with a major focus on neurofeedback, a treatment that is proving beneficial for children on the autism spectrum. Other promising treatments are also discussed.

Neurofeedback is a form of biofeedback that retrains the autistic brain to pay attention to the task at hand by rewarding attempts to focus. Research on autism shows that neurofeedback can remediate some abnormalities seen inside the brain, leading to overall symptom reduction and functional improvement. While helping them improve their social and communication skills, and gaining control over their behavior, neurofeedback can also help the underlying abnormal electrical activity seen in the brain of some people with autism (see Chapter 4). This abnormal electrical activity has been linked to seizures.

Neurofeedback and the Functioning of the Brain

The brain works through a combination of electrical and chemical activities that continuously influence each other. The electrical signals are transmitted at different speeds or frequencies, which help determine our mental state at any given moment. The brain waves can range from a low frequency, as seen during sleep (delta waves), to somewhat faster frequencies in semi-awake states (theta waves), to more relaxed states (alpha waves), to the highly alert state characterized by beta waves.

To perform any function, different parts of the brain have to communicate with each other. This happens when the electrical signals fire in synchrony with each other. At the same time, different regions perform independently because different parts of the brain have specific functions. While we want to see some parts function independently from the other areas, we want to see some parts of our brain's cortex maintain the normal level of independence.[84]

It has been found that in autism parts of the frontal lobes of the brain are often not working independently and are too connected, causing what is called a hyperconnectivity. *Hyperconnectivity* is used in medical terminology to explain billions and billions of nerve cells creating excessive connections, and this has been associated with epileptic seizures[85] in addition to schizophrenia.

Functional imaging studies of the brains of individuals who are diagnosed with ASD revealed neural connectivity problems that can be excessively high or low. It is important for all the parts of our brain to coordinate with the other parts for optimal functioning. Neurofeedback attempts to regulate brain waves by adjusting the degree of connectivity in different areas of the brain to approximate a more typical functioning brain, and this has shown a positive effect in reducing the symptoms of autism.

In one study using connectivity-guided neurofeedback, pre- and post-analysis showed a 40 percent reduction in autistic symptoms, enhancement of function between the brain and behavior, as well as a reduction of the hyperconnectivity.[86] This form of EEG biofeedback

---

84 *Neurofeedback guidelines for parents.* http://www.jacobsassociates.org/id25.html
85 *Hyperconnectivity.* http://en.wikipedia.org/wiki/Hyperconnectivity#cite_note_12#cite_note-12
86 *Neurofeedback helps.* http.sciencedaily.com/releases/2008/02/080226185848.htm

uses scalp EEG or FMRI (functional magnetic resonance imaging) to provide signals and send feedback about brain activity in real time.

Since 2000, Dr. Linden, a licensed clinical psychologist and the director of the Attention Learning Center in San Juan Capistrano, California, has been researching the efficacy of neurofeedback with autism. He has identified a hyperarousal in the brain activity in 50 percent of the subjects he studied.

Linden reports that approximately 33 percent of students with autism have abnormal EEG/seizure disorders, which can be seen on an EEG. But other seizures do not show up on EEGs. Dr. Linden agrees that although these mild, silent seizures often go unnoticed, they may significantly interfere with communication and behavior.

A review of multiple studies showed that the rate of abnormal EEGs in autism ranged from 10 to 83 percent, while the mean incidence was 50 percent. Atypical EEGs often predict poor outcomes for intelligence, speech, and educational achievement.[87]

In researching QEEG[88] brain mapping patterns of individuals with ASD, Linden found that QEEG-guided neurofeedback can normalize abnormal EEG/seizures and improve social skills, communication, over-focusing and attention problems.[89] "Our treatment is showing remarkable improvements in our patients with ASD, highlighted in the areas of behavior and attention. We have seen nonverbal patients with ASD begin to use language, increase eye contact and improve socialization," says Linden. "These are the most remarkable results we have seen in 20 years. The kids are developing a sense of humor, much to our and their parents' astonishment."

---

87 Hughes & John (1999).
88 A quantitative EEG (QEEG) is a computer analysis of the EEG signal.
89 Coben, Linden, & Myers (2010).

Researchers in this field have been examining patients with brain waves that consistently reveal abnormal EEGs. In particular, they frequently see too much beta activity in some of the brain waves of patients with ASD, causing the brain to overfocus. This overstimulation contributes to behaviors such as obsession, ritualism and anxiety.[90]

What Is a Neurofeedback Session Like?

Two computers are used: one for the patient and one for the clinician. Sensors are placed on the patient's scalp and ears to record the electrical activity of his brain waves. The brain waves are subsequently converted into signals that are transmitted to the clinician's computer. A picture of the electrical activity (EEG) is displayed for the clinician.

In the meantime, the patient is sitting in front of a computer that displays a game. The patient's brain waves prompt the game to begin. As the patient interacts with the game, he or she becomes aware of the different brain states or levels of attention, such as relaxed, daydreaming or alert. The clinician monitors the patient's EEG during each session and makes adjustments on his or her computer, which enables the patient to succeed at the game while retraining the brain waves.

While playing the computer game, patients are taught to recognize their brain wave pattern and regulate it. As the patient learns to control and improve his or her brain wave patterns, the game scores increase, thereby motivating progress.

Results of Neurofeedback

Reports indicate that "normalized" brain wave patterns lead to improvements in impulsive/hyperactive behavior and anxiety, together with increased attention, communication and socialization.[91]

90 Linden et al. (2010).
91 Linden et al. (2010).

Measurable IQ increases have also been seen, and the effects are long-lasting. This method is best used with children 4 years or older who are able to interact with the computer game. The technique is very safe and is done at least twice a week for a specified time period, depending upon the severity of the autism. On average, students with autism need 50-80 sessions, but preliminary results are typically seen after 10-15 sessions.[92]

Arlene Martell, a parent who has tried this treatment with her son, describes the experience in her online book, *Getting Adam Back: A Journey With Autism and Seizure.*

"Adam has epilepsy and autism. We began doing neurofeedback and all I can say is it was a new beginning. I began to notice significant changes in Adam. He was paying attention and learning new skills such as math. I did not tell his teachers, but soon after starting his teachers cornered me and wanted to know what changes have occurred with Adam. They were certain we had been doing something significant and were eager to learn what it was. Suddenly he was participating in class and making terrific progress."[93]

The biggest impacts were in the following areas:

- Major reduction in OCD (obsessive-compulsive disorder)
- Child's learning started again
- Reading level improved from grades 1 to 2
- Child began learning math
- More control over violent behavior
- Total reduction in seizures
- Child understood consequences
- Child was more aware of things going on around him

92 Linden et al. (2010).
93 Martell (2006).

- Child started to become more "normal"
- Child started to play with siblings
- Child spontaneously asked for things he wanted

"The doctor who administered 40 sessions was elated and could not believe the significant changes in him."[94]

Other Research Studies

Thompson and colleagues (2010) summarized data from a review of neurofeedback training with 150 patients diagnosed with Asperger Syndrome (AS) and 9 patients with ASD, who were seen over a period of 15 years in a clinical setting. The main objective was to examine if neurofeedback made a significant difference in patients diagnosed with AS. An additional aim was to provide practitioners with a detailed description of the method used to address some of the key symptoms in order to encourage further research and clinical work to refine the use of neurofeedback in individuals with AS and ASD.

Patients received 40-60 sessions, and for the most part, feedback was contingent upon decreasing the slow wave activity, decreasing beta spindling if it was present, and increasing fast wave activity. Metacognitive strategies relevant to social awareness, reading comprehension, math and spatial reasoning were taught when the feedback indicated that the patients were relaxed, calm, and focused.

Significant improvements were found on measures of attention. Scores on the Test of Variables of Attention (TOVA) and IQ rose 9 points, on average, as measured by the Wechsler Intelligent Scales. The decrease in AS symptoms coupled with measurable gains in IQ provides support for using neurofeedback as an effective treatment.[95]

---

94 A. Martell (personal communication, 2012).
95 Thompson, Thompson, & Reid (2010).

Case studies of neurofeedback trials with clients diagnosed with ASD have been reported for more than 15 years. Cowan and Markham[96] presented the first case study about an 8-year-old autistic girl with high-functioning ASD. Detecting high alpha and theta, predominantly in the parietal and occipital lobes of the brain, these researchers designed a protocol to suppress the inequalities noted.

After 21 sessions, the girl exhibited sustained attention, a decrease in her problem behaviors such as spinning and inappropriate giggling and a significant increase in her ability to attend to task. Her social skills also improved, based on parent and teacher reports. The TOVA,[97] which measures inattention and impulsivity, was administered before and after she received neurofeedback. She showed substantial improvement, which led to a normal result when the test was given two years later.

In the first controlled study of neurofeedback with individuals with ASD,[98] 12 children were each assigned to a control group. The experimental group received a mean of 36 treatment sessions. Treatment protocols were based on a standard protocol (not QEEG-based) to determine over-, under- and unstable arousal. The Autism Treatment Evaluation Checklist (ATEC), a free scoring instrument, was used to assess outcome.[99] Children who completed neurofeedback training attained an average of 26 percent reduction in the total ATEC-rated autism symptoms in contrast to 3 percent for the control group. Parents reported improvement in socialization, vocalization, anxiety, schoolwork, tantrums and sleep while the control group had minimal changes in these domains.

---

96 Cowan & Markham (1994).
97 http://www.tovatest.com/
98 Jarusiewicz (2002).
99 Rimland & Edelson (2000).

Another study of the effects of neurofeedback was conducted by Kouijzer et al. (2009).[100] Fourteen children with PDD-NOS (pervasive developmental disorder-not otherwise specified), 7 in the treatment and 7 in the waitlist (no treatment) control group, were matched for age, gender and intelligence, but were not randomly assigned. The treatment group received 40 sessions of neurofeedback treatment at scalp location C4. The study revealed that the neurofeedback-trained group demonstrated significant improvement in executive functioning, auditory attention, response inhibition, set-shifting and goal setting compared to the control group. Results of parent rating scales also showed improvements in social interaction, communication and typical behavior.

The largest published research to date of neurofeedback for ASD studied 49 children on the autism spectrum.[101] The experimental group included 37 children who received QEEG connectivity-guided neurofeedback (20 sessions performed twice per week); the control group included 12 children, who were matched for age, gender, race, handedness, treatments received and severity of ASD. A broad range of assessments was utilized, including parental judgment of outcome, neuropsychological tests, behavior rating scales, QEEG analysis and infrared imaging. Based on parental judgment of outcome, there was an 89 percent success rate for neurofeedback. In particular, there was an average 40 percent reduction in core ASD symptomology. There were also significant improvements, compared to the control group, on neuropsychological measures of attention, executive functioning, visual-perceptual processes and language functions. Reduced cerebral hyperconnectivity was associated with positive clinical outcomes in this population. The researchers reported that neurofeedback with ASD had a 91:1 benefit-harm ratio, a ratio of students having positive changes compared to

100 Kouijer, de Moor, Gerrits, Buitelaar, & Van Schie (2009).
101 Coben & Padolsky (2007).

negative side effects. This was by far the highest ratio of any other treatment for ASD ever studied.[102]

Major Improvements Noted as a Result of Neurofeedback Treatment

- Sustained attention
- Improved grades
- Improved sleep
- Enhanced communication and language
- Reduction in problematic behaviors
- Improved EEG patterns and seizure activity
- Higher IQ scores
- Reduced impulsivity and hyperactivity
- Decreased anxiety and over-focusing
- Improved social skills

Other Treatment Options

We conclude this chapter by looking at other treatments that are increasingly being found effective for addressing autism and seizure symptoms.

Specialized/Behavior Modification

Dr. Miranda has observed that neuronal connections are created and then reinforced through behavior modification techniques or applied behavior analysis and uses them at his clinic in addition to medication. During such treatments the patients practice, study and reinforce what they learn.

---

102 Coben & Padolsky (2007).

According to Dr. Miranda, "We can try to repair some of the problems in the central nervous system, but therapies designed to meet a child's specific needs are essential to enable effective learning to continue. Then it is prudent to use EEG and MRI as biomarkers, which would measure the level of recovery after treatment has commenced." Dr. Miranda has observed significant neuronal growth following targeted efficacious training in areas of the brain that previously showed atrophy.[103] Not only are measurable gains seen in behavioral improvements, they can also be measured by clinical testing.

Diet

A ketogenic diet has been used successfully to reduce the frequency of seizures in some patients with epilepsy, but the exact mechanism is not fully understood. Consisting of a reduced-protein and carbohydrate diet with an emphasis on a higher fat intake, it creates the metabolic state known as "ketosis," which is when the body breaks down fat and uses it for energy. It is a very strict diet implemented under the supervision of a neurologist.

I have known parents who credit this diet with their child's recovery from seizures. Josh has benefited from a low-sugar diet with an emphasis on fresh fruits and vegetables.

According to Donna Williams, "For me, l-glutamine has helped to lower the inflammatory processes. Omega 3 fatty acids keep my moods together and help me reduce over-stimulation. Calcium-magnesium and zinc seem to help with mood, sleep, digestion, and stress. Gluten-free and casein-free help me, and I rotate foods to avoid allergic response. Epilepsy and autism are single words ... but they are different ... and there are many underlying conditions in each of us to be discovered."[104]

---

103 F. Miranda (personal communication, May 5, 2009).
104 Williams. (2010).

Medication

A medication may lessen the number of seizures, but certain seizure types are considered refractory to treatment (that is, they are difficult to completely control).[105] Seeking a therapeutic dose (a dose that produces either a cessation or a reduction in symptoms) will require patience and a team effort between you and your child's physician. Sometimes a second medication is needed to control certain types of seizures.

Dr. Manuel Casanova, a prominent neuroscientist researcher in autism, shared some of his insights about the brain and another treatment that might be helpful.

Most researchers accept that autism is a condition of the brain that originates before a patient is born. By the time of puberty, one third of patients with ASD will have exhibited at least two unprovoked seizures.[106] Anecdotal case reports have shown that anticonvulsants have improved autistic traits in epileptic patients. More recently, an open trial of Depakote (an anticonvulsant) showed that patients sustained improvement in core symptoms and associated features, including affective instability, impulsivity and aggression.

Alternatively, another non-medication approach might be helpful in all suspected cases of seizure. There is a new potential therapy called repetitive transcranial magnetic stimulation (RTMS) that may help the seizure condition associated with autism. RTMS offers a noninvasive method for altering excitability of the brain. Seizures represent the extreme in cortical excitability, and RTMS potentially induces a short-term reorganization of the human

---

105 N. Minshew (personal communication, June 4, 2008).
106 M. Casanova (personal communication, April 2, 2009).

cortex. Neurological and psychological test results and brain ac-
tivity measurements tell us that RTMS helps with the symptoms
that people with autism find most distressing. The method cre-
ates a low-frequency magnetic field that pulses around the pa-
tient's brain through a coil placed on the scalp. It creates an elec-
trical current that enhances the performance of certain cells that
protect the brain from too much sensory input. RTMS is simple to
perform, inexpensive, and considered safe.

Autism is a developmental disorder. This means that the symp-
toms develop at an early age and often do not improve much
over time. The end result of this brain dysfunction is an inability to
filter out the extraneous information in our world, almost akin to
"feeling everything and hearing everything. Looking at a person's
face is like looking at the sun. You must squint your eyes to focus
on the particulars. This makes social interaction difficult if not im-
possible. In some cases the amplification of the signals provides
for seizures. Therefore, an early intervention is needed to achieve
the maximum therapeutic effect.

We have focused on using our new understanding of the brain
function to treat autism instead of only using medication to re-
mediate its consequences.[107]

In addition to the medications available to treat seizures, the treatments discussed in this chapter hold great promise. New discoveries are happening at lightning speed, so it is important to stay up on
new findings and be ready to discuss them with your child's team.
As emphasized throughout this book, it is important to work with
qualified professionals and not take claims of "cure" and efficacy at
face value.

---

107 M. Casanova (personal communication, April 2, 2009).

CHAPTER 8

FAMILY STORIES

Several families graciously offered to share their unique experiences with seizures in the context of autism.

Samuel's Story

Having a child with extreme special needs places a parent in unique situations throughout their lives. There are many hard-fought battles, but the appreciation of the joys is that much more precious. My son (now 16) began life as a typical baby. He was beautiful, outgoing and charming, reaching most of the milestones his first year. He learned to put two or three words together before the age of 14 months, such as "go to car," "where'd it go?" "see cat," and so on.

But suddenly at 15 months, he became completely silent. Soon after that he stopped understanding words we said to him, and was unable to follow the simplest of directions.

This was the beginning of this journey, and our lives changed completely the day he was diagnosed with autism. Many of the skills he'd already learned began to disappear. He would sing, for example, whole songs with words, and the following week they were gone. It was nearly unbearable to see my son disappearing before my eyes. He became nonverbal just after 2 years old and remains so today.

From the first day of his diagnosis, he had intense 1:1 teaching much of his waking hours. We tried "floor time,"[108] ABA,[109] as well as TEACCH.[110]

There was often no progress; in fact, Samuel continued to regress. Small incidents of aggression started to emerge at age 6. I believed that this was mostly due to his exceptionally poor communication skills, but the episodes were random. He could be in the same classroom with the same triggers and challenges and do fine for many days, and then suddenly he would lash out for seemingly no reason. His teachers – and I too – found it easy to dismiss this by calling it "acting out" or "having a bad day like everyone else has," but it became disturbing as he grew older, stronger and more violent, with no pattern to his aggression.

The ABA program he attended documented everything – every possible trigger or antecedent – such as too much stimulation, too little, too much pressure, too little, too noisy in the classroom, too quiet, etc. After years of data keeping, still no pattern emerged. The only pattern was that there was no pattern, no clear trigger. The behaviors were episodic.

My son was deteriorating before my eyes. At age 10, he began developing self-injurious behaviors. His acts of aggression and self-injurious behaviors were so severe that I was afraid he would hurt himself and others to the point of hospitalization or worse. I became increasingly desperate as nothing was helping. We ended up numerous times in our local crisis center, and he consequently lost his day

---

108 Floor time is a specific therapeutic technique designed to meet the child at his developmental level and building of the child's strengths. Therapy is often done on the floor by engaging in play activities. http://www.autismspeaks.org/what-autism/treatment/floortime-dir

109 ABA (applied behavior analysis) is the science of human behavior. It is the design, implementation, and evaluation of environmental modifications to produce socially significant improvement and behavior. ABA uses the tools of direct observation, measurement, and functional analysis of the relationship between the environment and behavior. It focuses upon the external environment to explain behavior rather than the internal constructs that are beyond our control. While this method has its merits, it completely disregards the possibility that behavior can be a consequence of something medical, such as a seizure. http://www.shapingbehavior.com/whatisaba.html

110 TEACCH (Treatment and Education of Autistic and Related Communication-Handicapped Children) tries to respond to the needs of people with autism using the best available approaches with a goal of obtaining the highest level of independence possible. The major thrust is to obtain the highest level of communication. Http://www.autism-resources.com/papers/TEACCHN.htm

school placement. We met with various doctors, behaviorists and naturopaths. My son was on a plethora of medications.

In this state, about a year ago, I read Caren's [Haines] research notes and identified immediately with her testimonials of how much improvement her son Josh had made, as well as the doctors' descriptions of temporal lobe seizures. I realized then that this is what was happening to my son, too! These acts of violence were not environmental behaviors, but the result of seizures that were causing him extreme distress. I was sure of it.

We have since followed a medical protocol that treats the episodes as seizures and the associated psychosis. Samuel is now in his seventh month without any severe episodes. His home school teacher had never seen him focus for two hours straight in all the years she had worked with him. Now within the past month, he has made an incredibly smooth transition to a residential school about three hours from home. Thanks to finally being on the proper medications, he has adapted to his new life, able to attend and focus in the classroom, share a bedroom with another boy, share a house with six other boys and participate in a variety of activities in the community. I talk with his aides each evening, and they report that he rarely stops smiling. They say he is "charming and outgoing."

I think back and remember that this is the way he was before he was diagnosed. His true personality can once again shine through. It is amazing to me that he can now live away from the rest of his family and is capable of creating a life of his own. My thrill at finding this incredible book, and finally being able to bring peace to this child, and to know that he can look forward to a future of value and dignity, nearly defies words.

Michael's Story

Michael was an easy and happy baby until we began to notice a change at around 15 months of age. One day as I was next to him while he played with his blocks in bed, I was startled to realize that the bed was shaking. I looked over at him and saw his hands were shaking and his lips were bluish. As I tried to speak with him, I noticed he was just staring. Soon afterwards, he fell into a deep sleep.

I immediately called Mike's doctor, and we made an appointment to have an EEG. It didn't show any seizure activity, so no further action was taken. Over the next eight months, Mike's behavior became very erratic while he exhibited many unexplained temper tantrums and I continued to see what I considered to be seizure activity.

When I called his doctor to report my concern, I felt he was minimizing my observations and treating me as if I knew little about such issues. He gave me a list of things to do in terms of behavior management, which I continued to try, all the while watching Mike's behavior go from bad to worse. He was kicking, biting, hitting and screaming on a daily basis. He became upset for no apparent reason, and I felt clueless to understand it and powerless to help him.

What was I overlooking? What could I have done to make him so upset? I was searching for answers that just led to more questions. I felt guilty when family members weighed in with their assessment of our situation, claiming, "He is just spoiled."

I couldn't imagine how that could be. It wasn't *our* behavior that was changing; it was *his*. Of course, I examined my own behavior, but always came up empty. I tried to enroll my son in daycare to see if things would change. I knew they wouldn't "spoil" him there, and I hoped separating from me would be good for him. But the daycare was constantly calling me to say that Mike was engaging in unacceptable behaviors, such as biting other children. I felt embarrassed, but at the same time I realized that their behavior management techniques also seemed to "spoil" him.

I continued to see what I was certain was seizure activity, but all of my observations were discounted as my son continued his downward spiral. Attempting to come up with solutions, the staff of the preschool he attended so many years ago suggested that they call in their psychologist. When I met with him, he said that from my description and his observations, it sounded like temporal lobe seizures. He put me in touch with a child development facility and, based upon his assessment, an appointment was made.

Michael displayed all the behaviors that were of concern during this lengthy evaluation, yet the experts disagreed on whether any of this could be seizure-related. Tourette Syndrome seemed to garner the therapeutic consensus, and an antipsychotic, Haldol, was prescribed. But there was no improvement, and I continued to observe the behavior, which I considered to be seizure-related.

A special preschool was recommended when he turned 3, and it was decided that Mike would attend five mornings a week. The purpose was to integrate children with behavior problems into a class with typically behaving peers.

The other children continued to progress as we watched Michael continue to regress. If he were pushed to complete tasks, he would have temper tantrums that seemed purposeful at times. During these bouts of unprovoked rage, he destroyed everything in sight. Interesting, at times he would suddenly stop and say "Mickey's a good boy; good boys don't bite, good boys don't hit," etc. He knew all the right things to do and would try to tell us that he was good, but he just could not control himself.

The current team suggested that he be evaluated at the local psychiatric institute and clinic. He was turning 4, and nothing had helped him thus far. During the initial evaluation, I conveyed all of the incidents that seemed to me to be seizure activity. The staff wished to have a opportunity to evaluate this possibility, which required a lengthy stay of approximately one week, but would be important in the overall scheme.

I was told that Mike didn't seem to be having seizures. Later I found out this was not true; to the contrary, a wonderful team of doctors were indeed seeing seizure activity and were relaying this to Mike's "in charge" physicians.

Dr. Nancy Minshew and Dr. James Payton, who were staff doctors at that time, told another doctor in charge of Michael's case that they thought he was having seizures and that he needed to be treated accordingly. It felt like a conspiracy was going on. Only later did I realize that there was a discrepancy and that the "in charge" doctor was omitting segments of what he was being told. I will never know why.

After Mike's release, I took him to the clinic to see Drs. James Payton and Nancy Minshew, and soon after he began to embark on another sort of journey ... wellness! His bouts of seizure continued as we waited patiently for the appointment date to arrive. There were times we noticed that "the lights were on, but no one was home." The slightest thing would set him off when this occurred – at one point, he tried to throw the kitchen chair through a window. I wrestled him to the floor to keep him from hurting himself, not realizing that he had an orange marker in his hand. After the episode, he had no idea how he or I got orange marks all over us. He was surprised and perplexed. He didn't know what happened, why or how.

Under Dr. Minshew's care, we finally got his seizures under control. This was not easy, but wrought with many ups and downs, since determining optimal dosing of the medication takes time and patience. Precision is the goal, which has a price attached. Too little and he is seizing, too much and he is sleeping all day. Thank heaven for doctors who continue to "get it and then get it right."

Evan's Story

I did not initially understand that Evan was suffering from seizures, but I knew something was amiss. When Evan turned 2, I began to notice frequent episodes where my son would stop an activity and just stare into space. On a few occasions, he also displayed facial grimacing, eyes rolling back and blinking rapidly.

Luckily, a neurologist at the most prominent autism center in the country formally diagnosed Evan's seizures when they fortunately showed up on an EEG, so we didn't have the years of suffering many families go through with this diagnosis. Evan was given an overnight EEG, which showed he had partial epileptic seizures originating from the right parietal lobe, which would then generalize to the left lobe.

Once seizure medication began, he had many fewer seizures, although he still seized from time to time. He would exhibit eye rubbing, eyes rolling, shivering and facial grimaces, and he would become unresponsive for a minute after exhibiting these symptoms. Depakote was ordered for him, and it was helping since we noted there were fewer bouts, but the episodes were still occurring, leading us to wonder if his dose was too low or if he simply had refractory epilepsy.[111]

---

111 Some experts define a patient as having refractory seizures if treatment fails to achieve seizure freedom for 12 months or more.

Evan's seizures affected his behavior and his early development. He was delayed in many areas, including his gross- and fine-motor skills and verbal communication. He was a passive baby approaching one year of age and would just play quietly with the same toy for hours. His eye contact was absent, which was a concern, and we sought to have a neurological evaluation to explain the conglomeration of symptoms we were seeing.

He was diagnosed with mild autism by the neurologists at the same center where he had his initial EEG testing. He was later placed into an intensive applied behavior analysis program. He did well though he continued to suffer from symptoms of seizure until we got the medication dosage adjusted correctly. That took a bit of time.

Evan started to acquire more words, and his communication got noticeably better as the Depakote was brought to a more therapeutic level. His autism symptoms have improved significantly since we began treating his seizures, and miraculously, he has been able to be included in general education classes with typical peers. We are very lucky that his seizures showed up on an EEG and that, consequently, he was treated early.

Stories such as these are echoed all over the world every single day as we learn more and more about the association of developmental problems, intellectual disability and the high correlation with seizure. We are trying to learn where one begins and another ends as we sift through the pages of abstracts, case studies, articles and family stories. If we begin to ask more questions, the answers might just follow.

CHAPTER 9

A PSYCHIATRIST'S VIEW

By Darold A. Treffert, MD
Clinical Professor, Department of Psychiatry,
University of Wisconsin Medical School

Every sophomore class at the University of Wisconsin Medical School was greeted by the distinguished and revered white-haired surgery professor in the same way. He would ask the students, one by one: "What's the treatment for the common cold?"

Eager students, including myself, would put forth suggestions: Decongestants? Aspirin? Acetaminophen? Cough drops? Antibiotics? Aerosols? Each answer was routinely met with a resounding "No" from the professor.

After exhausting the lengthy list (and the class), the professor made this pronouncement: "The first step in treatment is to make a diagnosis. Before you reach for a remedy or the prescription pad, be sure you have made the correct diagnosis." And he is right! The first step in treatment *is* to make a diagnosis.

The professor then continued, "And how do you make that diagnosis? Remember – always remember – to *listen to the patient,* because he or she is giving you the answer. Instead of immediately ordering and then relying on lab work, X-rays or whatever more exotic tests you might order, the first order of business is to *listen to the patient,* because he or she is giving you the diagnosis. And if you missed it the first time around, listen again, only this time listen more carefully."

The professor is right on both scores. The first step in treatment is to make a diagnosis, and we make the diagnosis by listening to the patient. Those were the two most valuable lessons I learned in medical school, and I put them to immediate use when a 45-year-old woman was admitted to the psychiatric unit and I was assigned her case. She had come to the hospital voluntarily at the request of her family. They were concerned because she had gained a great deal of weight, had lost interest in her work and home, had slipped in her grooming and personal habits and was generally very depressed. The family was worried because the depression was deep and was atypical for this woman – their wife and mother.

I took a history, which included a detailed "review of systems," which, as a beginning resident, I was still inclined to do (today I must confess my review of systems is more hurried and often not quite so compulsively detailed thanks to years of experience). I asked about each of the cranial nerves, one by one. When I asked whether her sense of smell had changed at all she said, "Funny you should ask that. This last weekend we were going up to the cottage and we put the outboard motor in the trunk of the car as we always do. I saw that the gas cap on the motor was loose and some gasoline was leaking into the car trunk, but I didn't smell the gas, which seemed rather odd. But until just now when you asked if I had noticed any changes in my ability to smell things, I had forgotten about it."

To make a long clinical story short, this patient's loss of smell was the clue to a search for an organic cause of her symptoms. It turns out she had a benign midline meningioma.[112] The tumor was surgically removed, and her sense of smell returned, her appetite lessened, her mood lifted and she quickly returned to "her old self," much to her relief and the relief of her grateful family.

---

112 Meningioma is one of the most common benign brain tumors.

Another patient came to that same service under my care. He too was middle-aged but with a very different complaint. He had abruptly lost his hearing, *entirely,* about two months earlier with no accompanying symptoms. He was put through an extensive and expensive work-up on the ENT (ear, nose and throat) service, where it was determined that the hearing apparatus, including nerve testing, was intact. Because there was no apparent organic basis for the hearing loss, the patient was transferred to the psychiatric service, since it was thought that his symptom must be "all in his head."

Since he couldn't hear, I had to correspond with him via written notes. After quite a long time using this technique, I remembered that sophomore class advice ... *Listen to the patient.* So I wrote a note asking, "Why do *you* think you can't hear?" "Because I don't have any ears," he wrote back. "If you don't have any ears, you can't hear."

It turns out this gentleman had selectively hallucinated his ears away in what is called a *nihilist delusion* or *negation delusion.* Patients with that disorder can selectively, negatively hallucinate away, as it were, a limb, organ or other body part. For them, when they look in the mirror, whatever body part has been deluded away simply doesn't exist. And, of course, if you don't have ears, how can you hear?

A few days and a few milligrams of an antipsychotic later, the patient's ears returned, and he could hear again. His nihilist delusion disappeared, and his ears returned to their natural spot.

It would have been so much simpler, and less expensive, if one of the ENT residents had simply asked the patient, "Why do *you* think you can't hear?" Like my wise professor advised, "Listen to the patient, he's giving you the diagnosis."

I routinely ask my patients and their families, "What do *you* think is going on here?" You would be surprised how often their assessment is informative and critical. In many ways, the patients know themselves best, as do their families. So for me, taking a family history is more than just listing past family illnesses. It is also about asking the families for their observations and input, which is so often very valuable and insightful.

Psychomotor Epilepsy and the Psychiatric Patient

Later in my residency, I did a clinical rotation at what was then called the Diagnostic Center in Madison, Wisconsin. It was a state-operated outpatient facility for comprehensive, multidisciplinary evaluations of children and adolescents. I was intrigued with a subset of patients, whose main symptom and reason for referral was "rage episodes," sometimes with rather severe aggression. The EEGs in these patients often showed a particular paroxysmal spike and wave pattern for what was then called "14 and 6 thalamic or hypothalamic epilepsy." These clinical episodes of rage were abrupt and seizure-like in character, but not associated with overt grand mal or any other seizure patterns. These patients sparked my interest in the relationship between EEG findings and the psychiatric patient, particularly in the absence of overt seizures.

So in 1964 I carried out a study entitled "The Psychiatric Patient With an EEG Temporal Lobe Focus " to assess how often what were in fact, epileptic disorders (psychomotor epilepsy) were diagnosed as psychiatric disorders.

In the paper, I wanted to point out how, with this group of patients in particular, neurology and psychiatry merged into the field of neuropsychiatry. I pointed out that the incidence of serious psychiatric disturbance in other forms of epilepsy is as low as 10 percent, whereas in patients with psychomotor epilepsy, earlier studies had reported that as many as 40 percent had psychiatric disturbances, and a third of those were disturbed enough to be psychotic.[113]

---

113 Gibbs (1958, pp. 278-294).

I summarized the literature up to that point, which had shown, while diversified, that a number of types of behaviors had come to be associated with temporal lobe epilepsy (TLE), including aggression, catatonia, fugue states,[114] amnesia, depersonalization, déjà vu, hallucinations, sudden mood changes and panic attacks, to name only some.

I also pointed out that "whether one chooses to call it psychomotor epilepsy or not, the finding of temporal lobe spiking occurs in about 8-10 percent of the unselected psychiatric population, and in certain groups – aggressive and catatonics – the incidence rises to 25 percent. It is likely to be associated with paroxysmal, episodic symptoms that include catatonic furor, combativeness, black-outs, hallucinations, and uncontrolled aggression. *Often the psychiatric symptoms so dominate the clinical picture that the ictal[115] quality of the symptoms is overlooked and, on the basis of symptoms more familiar to the psychiatrist, the patient is given a conventional psychiatric diagnosis."[116]*

For my study, I compared 17 adult psychiatric patients who did show an EEG abnormality (anterior temporal lobe spiking) with 17 patients matched for age, sex and psychiatric diagnoses without EEG abnormality.[117] Results showed that patients with anterior temporal lobe spiking demonstrated much more in the way of aggressive behaviors and episodic symptoms than those with identical psychiatric diagnoses but no EEG abnormality. In spite of identical psychiatric diagnoses, the group without temporal lobe spiking showed much more in the way of classic psychiatric symptoms such as delusions and thought disorder. In short, the group of patients with temporal lobe spiking looked more "epileptic" than "psychotic."

---

114 A rare psychiatric disorder characterized by reversible amnesia for personal identity, including the memories, personality and other identifying characteristics of individuality. Anand (2005): Autism and epilepsy: The complex relationship between cognition, behavior, and seizure. *The Internet Journal of Neurology* 4(1).
115 Seizure-like.
116 Treffert (1964, emphasis added).
117 Treffert (1964).

Temporal Lobe Epilepsy: The Great Pretender

This study demonstrated that temporal lobe spiking on the EEG in a group of patients with psychiatric diagnoses – even in the absence of overt epilepsy – has clinical psychiatric significance, and that the clinician, whether a neurologist or a psychiatrist, must be fully aware of this overlap between psychiatry and neurology in such patients.

One does this by carefully listening to the patient and being fully aware that sometimes TLE can "pretend" to be a number of unrelated disorders and can present as psychosis, panic attacks, rage, hallucinations, sudden mood changes and catatonia, to name only some of the more common.

I am neither alone nor original in pointing out the hazards of the difficult "hinterland" between psychiatry and neurology with these patients. Thirty years later, further research pointed out that TLE "straddles the borderland between psychiatry and neurology" and that because TLE can present as disorders of thought, mood, or emotion, these patients often come to the attention of psychiatrists. But because these symptoms often exist in the absence of generalized grand mal seizures, "physicians may often fail to recognize the epileptic origin of the disorder. Indeed, misdiagnosis and failures of diagnosis are common."[118]

Since a variety of emotions can be triggered by temporal lobe dysfunction and can arise with no identifiable precipitant, an incorrect diagnosis of acute panic attack, for example, may be made.[119] Often overlooked, unless carefully elicited, is the *epileptic* nature of the events and the fact that such episodes are often accompanied by a "strong visceral component" and a sensation usually traveling from stomach to head in a "wave" fashion.

118 Restak (1995, p. 9).
119 Restak (1995).

These details are not immediately apparent and must be discovered via careful questioning and, as my medical school professor pointed out, listening to the patient. In the field of medicine, generally, this kind of questioning is referred to as a high "index of suspicion."

Panic Attack or Seizure?

For a number of conditions, the differential diagnosis between a psychiatric disorder and TLE is difficult and depends on a high index of suspicion. The fact that TLE and some psychiatric conditions can co-exist makes it all the more difficult. Space doesn't permit an exploration of all such circumstances, but looking at one of the most common overlapping conditions (and the newer methods available to help make a differential diagnosis) will provide a good example of such complexity.

Epilepsy and panic disorder are both common conditions. Lifetime prevalence of epilepsy is 3-4 percent; prevalence of panic disorder is 1 percent. The difficulty – and importance – of differentiating partial seizures and panic disorder is due to the overlap of symptoms.[120] In one study,[121] it was reported that panic disorder is the most common condition that needs to be distinguished from seizure disorders, 40 percent of which are TLE. This study includes detailed reports of five patients whose symptoms were initially felt to be psychiatric in origin and were treated as such. Only months later, after a high index of suspicion and careful workup, the true cause of their "panic disorder" was determined to be TLE, which responded well to anticonvulsant medication, which is neurologic rather than psychiatric (anti-anxiety) treatment.

There are references to a number of other papers wherein what was first thought to be panic disorder proved to be TLE and the overlap-

---

120 Thompson, Duncan, & Shelagh (2000).
121 Young et al. (1995, pp. 352-357).

ping characteristics of these two conditions.[122] The following provides some guidance for distinguishing those two conditions:

- Panic attacks are generally longer in duration than seizures.

- Ictal episodes are more stereotyped than panic attacks.

- While TLE might present initially with fear and anxiety, those feelings may progress to more classic organic symptoms such as olfactory auras or smells, amnesic features such as memory lapses, visceral accompaniments such as an odd feeling in the stomach or automatisms, which resembled repetitive movement. (TLE is more likely when the classic, more organic symptoms precede the panic feelings.)

- EEGs show that temporal lobe spiking panic attacks are more likely to occur with agoraphobia (fear of being in places where escape might be difficult or impossible).

- Positive family history occurs more commonly in panic disorder (as high as 25 percent).

Obviously when the source of the "panic attacks" is TLE rather than panic disorder, there are tremendous treatment implications. One study[123] describes a case in which a patient had three psychiatric hospital admissions in three months for "anxiety attacks." EEG and MRI findings were normal, but because the constellation of symptoms suggested temporal lobe epilepsy, a TLE diagnosis was considered and the patient responded rapidly and dramatically to anticonvulsant medication. The authors concluded that "panic disorder and temporal lobe epilepsy can be confused with each other; proper diagnosis is necessary for the selection of effective pharmacotherapy."

The point is that a high index of suspicion, careful listening to the

---

122 Hurley, Fisher, & Taber (2006, pp. 436-443).
123 Deutsch, Rosse, Sud, & Burket (2009, pp. 160-162).

patient and a comprehensive epilepsy workup are required in the frequent overlap in symptoms between temporal lobe epilepsy and panic disorder. While these conditions can co-exist in the same patient, careful diagnostic observations combined with EEG and imaging studies can separate them from each other, with obvious and critical treatment implications.

Epilepsy, Complex Partial Seizures and Autism Spectrum Disorders

Epileptic seizures occur frequently in individuals with ASD, with most reports putting that figure as high as 30-40 percent. One study reported clinical seizures in 41 percent of 78 children with autism.[124] Another found 40 percent of 56 patients with autism to have had epilepsy, and that the higher the impairment in the autism spectrum disorder, the higher the rate of epilepsy.[125] Tuchman, Cuccaro, and Alessandri[126] provide a comprehensive review of the history of autism and epilepsy linking a higher level of impairment to a higher chance of seizures. They have noted the same general correlation: The more severe the autism impairment, the higher the chance of seizures. Such seizure activity tends to occur in two different peaks – early childhood prior to age 5 and adolescence after age 10.

In patients with ASD who have demonstrable seizures, the vast majority of those events are partial complex seizures rather than grand mal seizures. One study followed 130 patients with "autistic disorder or atypical autism" for more than 10 years. Thirty-three patients in that group, or 26 percent, exhibited epileptic seizures, of which 61 percent were partial complex seizures and 39 percent were generalized seizures.[127] The age of onset of epilepsy ranged from 8 to 26 years.

124 Hughes & Melyn (2005, pp. 15-20).
125 Gabis, Pomeroy, & Andriola (2005).
126 (2010).
127 Hara (2007, pp. 486-490).

Adding to the difficulty of differential diagnosis is the fact that while children with generalized or partial complex seizures have abnormal EEGs to document the disorder, as many as 19 percent can have EEG abnormalities without clinical seizures.[128]

What are the symptoms or behaviors that are likely to raise that index of suspicion regarding the co-existence of autism and epilepsy? These include a history of regression in language, repetitive abnormal movements or behaviors with or without altered consciousness, staring episodes and episodic events of temper tantrums, or rage.[129] Such paroxysmal events deserve investigation regarding an ictal basis (epileptic). Beyond that, routine EEGs are advised for children who are low functioning or severely impaired, because a history of potential epileptic symptoms is more difficult to accurately ascertain in that group.

With respect to doing an EEG as a routine part of a workup of a patient with autism, researchers advise that there is little support for performing routine EEG in higher functioning children in the autism spectrum without significant symptoms suggestive of epilepsy, and without regression of language and communication.

In patients where clinical epilepsy is a co-existing condition, anticonvulsant therapy must be considered. Choice of such drugs will depend on the type of epilepsy seen. In instances in which an epileptic component has been identified as a contributing factor to the overall clinical picture in a patient with ASD, selecting the right medication in the right dose, on the right time schedule and in the right form can be a very delicate journey. Side effects of the anticonvulsants can be troublesome and intensify some of the autistic symptoms. Contrariwise, use of certain psychotropic medications

128 Hughes & Melyn (2005, pp. 15-20).
129 Gabis, Pomeroy, & Andriola (2005, pp. 652-656).

to control some specific disruptive or interfering behaviors in persons with ASD can increase seizure activity. This is where choice and dosage of medications directed to both the autism and the epilepsy becomes as much an art as a science. Experience dictates that doses start at very low levels, observation be diligent, choices be flexible, inventiveness be encouraged and patience prevail.

Landau-Keffler Syndrome

In the clinical scenarios above, psychomotor epilepsy can masquerade as panic attacks or seizures and can co-exist with ASD. But it is important to recognize that there is a separate form of epilepsy that produces autistic-*like* symptoms and behaviors, but is *not* a part of ASD. It is a disorder separate from autism and needs to be approached as such. Therefore, it deserves special mention and consideration.

In 1957, Landau and Keffler reported six cases of children who had developed typically, including language acquisition, but quite abruptly experienced loss of language with other major regression and autistic-*like* behaviors. Since that time, several hundred cases have been reported in the literature, making it still a rather rare condition. That disorder is now generally known as *acquired epileptic aphasia*[130] (see p. 31).

Children with this disorder have many autistic-*like* symptoms and, therefore, it is frequently misdiagnosed as autism, when in fact it is a convulsive disorder. Clinical seizures are present in 70-75 percent of patients, but all such patients, whether with clinical seizures or not, have EEG abnormalities consisting of high-amplitude (amplitude refers to the strength of the signal, how high it peaks and how low the brain waves travel compared to a straight line), spike

---

130 Landau & Keffler (1957, pp. 523-530).

and wave discharges (a pattern of brain wave seen in some types of epilepsy, this pattern is transient and clearly distinguishable from background activity with certain peaks, followed by waves), multi-focal or generalized. In some cases, only a sleep record divulges those abnormalities.

Typically, symptoms of Landau-Keffler Syndrome begin between the ages of 3 and 7, although they may begin as late as age 14. They can begin gradually or can occur following a first-time seizure. The child who had been developing normally begins to have difficulty understanding what is said (auditory agnosia), followed by difficulty replying (aphasia), which can lead to loss of language entirely. In beginning stages, many parents believe the child is deaf, and there are often accompanying behavioral changes. These latter two symptoms frequently lead to a suspicion of autism, since "suspected deafness" is a common accompaniment of autism, and behavioral changes abound. However, an EEG can be used to make the differential diagnosis.

CT (Cat scan) and MRI (magnetic resonance imaging) studies are usually normal and PET (positron emission tomography) studies have shown either unilateral or bilateral hypo- or hypermetabolism. (The brain metabolizes chemicals, which can be hypo-/under-used or hyper-/over-used, and this is seen in seizure disorders.) Microscopic examination of surgical specimens has shown minimal gliosis (accumulation of astrocytes in response to injury), but no evidence of encephalitis.

Treatment consists of anticonvulsants, speech therapy and, in some cases, steroids. This rare condition is mentioned here as a separate entity because the natural history of the disorder and its unique symptom complex overlap both autism and epilepsy. When those features are detected in a patient, it is important to realize that while there may be some autistic-like symptoms or behaviors, this condition is *not* an autism spectrum disorder. Instead, it is a seizure disorder and must to be treated as such.

The Epileptic Personality

In the epilepsy field overall, controversy continues as to whether there is or is not an "epileptic personality." In my 1964 temporal lobe study,[131] I summarized traits associated with epileptic personality as perseveration of thought and affect, circumstantiality, impulsiveness, irritability, pseudo-religiosity and paranoid tendencies.

In 1975, an article by Waxman and Geschwind[132] focused on the interictal[133] behavior of persons with temporal lobe epilepsy. This behavior included a combination of traits, such as deepened emotions, circumstantial thought, preoccupation with philosophical and religious beliefs and changes in sexual behavior. Eventually, that constellation of traits came to be known as the *Geschwind Syndrome*. Later studies[134] expanded Geschwind's observations to 18 behavioral traits that included mania, depression, guilt, humorlessness, altered sexual interest, aggression, anger and hostility, hypergraphia, religiosity, philosophical interest, sense of personal destiny, hypermoralism, dependency, paranoia, obsessionalism, circumstantiality and viscosity. Many of these same features are included in a number of psychiatric conditions and are not unique to temporal lobe epilepsy.[135]

---

131 Treffert (1964).
132 Waxman & Geschwind (1975).
133 Period of time between seizures.
134 Bear & Fedio (1977).
135 Barr (2003).

Seized – More to Explore

In 1993, Eve LaPlante wrote *Seized*.[136] It is a very reader-friendly book written in by a woman who has explored and summarized TLE comprehensively from historical, clinical and research standpoints. It tells the stories of several creative luminaries from the past who had TLE, including van Gogh, Dostoevsky, Tennyson, and Lewis Carroll, along with the detailed stories of some ordinary people, whose baffling symptoms were finally determined, after a circuitous route, to be TLE.

The book also provides a historical account of the major clinicians and researchers (Gastaut, Jackson, Penfield, Jasper, Geschwind) and their astute observations and elevated index of suspicion that led to important discoveries in the complex interface between body and mind that temporal lobe epilepsy presents. There are also chapters on diagnostic and intervention techniques, along with recent research efforts and findings, all written in easy-to-understand language.

I highly recommend this book for anyone wanting to know more about TLE. Interspersed liberally among the extensive information about TLE that this book provides, and shining throughout all its pages, is the tremendous empathy this author conveys for better understanding and supporting persons with TLE. That empathy and understanding provides a good role model for all of us and underscores the importance of "listening to the patient," which is where I began my journey with these persons in the first place.

Neurology + Psychiatry = Neuroscience

At the beginning of this chapter, I indicated that if ever there was an illness that by its very nature blends neurology and psychiatry into the specialty of neuropsychiatry, it is temporal lobe epilepsy. I would add

---

136 LaPlante (1993, 2000).

that autism is another such condition, as we are finding out that it likewise requires, of necessity, a clear understanding of both the brain and behavior. I have had a career-long interest in both.

Reflecting on where we are headed in the overlap between the brain and behavior, it seems to me that even the term *neuropsychiatry* is dated. Perhaps it would be better to name my specialty *neuroscience*, since a broader understanding of neuroscience overall is where the field is ultimately headed.

I, for one at least, am "blown away" by what is happening in neuroscience today. But one primary challenge remains, no matter what brand of specialty a doctor might apply to himself or herself – that is, no matter how startling the advances in science, the doctor must be as unfailingly interested in the patient who has the disease as he or she is interested in the disease the patient has. That's called *bedside manner*, and technology – no matter how shiny – must not detract from the delicate balance of caring *for* the patient and caring *about* him or her. Bedside manner and examining room techniques require "listening to the patient," as I have emphasized here. That simplicity will never vanish, no matter how sophisticated the technology.

CONCLUSION

Time literally stops, and life is nearly unlivable when a person and his family are besieged by the sudden uncontrollable rages and aggressive behaviors that can accompany a silent seizure disorder. The joy of living comes to a screeching halt as the family merely exists in survival mode. It is a living hell fraught with worry and unending strife. For many, as for my own family, this relentless reign of terror goes on every day for many years. The high incidence of seizure disorders seen in those diagnosed with autism would seem to indicate that some kind of anatomical brain abnormality is generating the unusual behaviors leading to the autism diagnosis.

It must be absolutely terrifying to be episodically driven to commit destructive behavior with no internal mechanism of control. In the midst of a seizure, a person loses touch so profoundly with the conscious world and has very little chance of being understood, which makes this scenario so utterly cruel. It is an overwhelming burden for the person who is suffering and for those who love and care for that person.

With the help of the dedicated physicians whose insights are shared throughout this book, I have found a way to treat my son successfully. Seizures can be vicious in their presentation; the associated behaviors are akin to a loss of brain control for those who experience them. Since these seizures mimic other brain abnormalities, the result is often chronic problems with misdiagnosis. The frequent association between epilepsy and psychosis needs exploration, in hopes of reaching a better understanding of this complicated condition and its many layers.

The very good news is that small miracles are occurring every single day in the world of autism. For some of the newly diagnosed on the autism spectrum, the miracle presents itself in the form of a child who loses the diagnosis and becomes indistinguishable from other children. For others, particularly older children whose seizures have gone undetected for some time, it can be a marked improvement in many critical areas of functioning and the children becoming the best they can be. Some people on the autism spectrum will live independently once they become adults, while others will need support and care for their entire lives. All of our children will have the best chance for success if we can identify and treat their underlying conditions accurately and as early in their development as possible.

Many parents are wondering why more research isn't being done on the connection between autism and seizures, especially since so many esteemed neurologists are telling us about autism's silent seizure connection. We need to look carefully at the constellation of behaviors exhibited in the form of autism and listen to what our children are telling us, either verbally or nonverbally. As concerned parents, we need to focus on the safe treatments that help many children with autism, such as ABA therapy, speech therapy, sensory integration, seizure medications, neurofeedback, gluten/casein-free diets, ketogenic diet and adding certain supplements if there is a deficiency. The day parents hear "your child has autism, which is a lifelong, debilitating condition," many begin a rapid descent into the grief process. Though we may try multiple interventions over the years with variable degrees of success, many of us have to face the reality of a very tough road with many ups and downs.

Underscoring some of the issues related to violent and difficult behaviors, we hear on the news about cases such as the one about the murder of a college professor. She was fleeing from a madman who was in a rage and appeared to be bent on killing her. She hid behind a door in her bedroom, but the door wasn't strong enough to protect her from his assault. She was viciously killed by her attacker. As we read a bit closer, we find that the perpetrator of this horrific crime was her 200-pound teenage son, diagnosed with autism as a young boy, who flew into blinding rage for no apparent reason. She had previously told colleagues her son was diagnosed with autism at a young age but that he was a sweetheart of a boy, who was episodically driven to commit violent attacks for no discernible reason.

This loving mother didn't know that the violent episodes that terrorized her by night might have been diagnosed as a treatable form of subclinical seizure if the science we rely upon had been more advanced. If she had known, maybe she could have prevented the terrible spiral down into the vortex of violence that seems to plague so many people afflicted by autism. It is sad she is not alive today to love and care for this vulnerable young man.

When I became desperate and despondent at the prospect that nothing would ever help my son, I felt forced to begin looking at residential placements. I was increasingly afraid of bodily harm and began to believe that I too might end up bruised, battered and perhaps dead. At that time I'd read about a mother who was repeatedly attacked by her son in random, similarly unprovoked episodes. She confessed to having many broken bones and diminished eyesight due to the relentless, episodic, unprovoked battery.

In desperation, she finally placed him in an institution because he became such a danger to her and her family. She recalled how he was sad and perplexed when she began to say goodbye to him, and how he looked at her with profound fear and panic when she began to walk to the door without him. She confided that this was by far the most painful moment of her life. When she got to her car, she began to sob uncontrollably, and she described being doubled over for hours, racked in pain and unable to drive. She said she remained in the parking lot of this residential placement for untold hours, alone in the depths of despair. It was brave of her to take this step. I personally could not have done it.

A few years ago while I was dealing with the worst rage behaviors, a friend called me. She began her conversation with, "I have great news."

Her son Jake, who is the same age as my son, Josh, had just received written news that he would get a basketball scholarship so he could attend the college of his dreams. His parents were understandably on top of the world.

What she did not know was that at the very moment she was telling me this, I was on my hands and knees on the floor wiping up small puddles of my own blood while pressing a bag of ice to my face. Only minutes earlier my son and I had been sharing a tender, loving exchange that turned dark in a matter of moments. I hung up the phone with my friend just as my son began to sob.

When we embarked on this road some 20 years ago, we desperately held onto the hope that our child on the spectrum would become one of the 50 percent who, we were led to believe, statistically could become indistinguishable from their peers through the rigors of 40-hour-per-week ABA therapy.[137] At that time, ABA was considered the major route with proven success. That ray of hope remained alive and well until the day my beautiful and loving child punched me with such force that it hurled me to my knees.

---

137 *About Lovaas. ABA for autism.* www.thelovaascenter.org

In Chapter 1, I described the day when Josh asked me to help him "fix" his brain. I feel fortunate that, through my extensive research and my intense belief in the knowledge that his troubling behaviors were not within his control, I now have come to understand that many of the underlying issues he faces such as seizure, psychosis and sleep disturbance can be remedied with medication.

His plea prompted my in-depth study of this issue, which has proven to be a very worthwhile endeavor. His brain function has greatly improved with the addition of the right combination of medications targeting seizure and psychosis. He is no longer exhibiting serious aggressive behavior; however, because we lost so many precious years without proper diagnosis and treatment, he now enters adulthood with a chronic psychosis in tow.

While it is compelling to know how frequently autism and seizure co-exist invisibly, this protocol may not work in every case of a person diagnosed with autism. This information is valuable in that it might help and, therefore, should be shared with parents of children diagnosed with autism and the professionals who work with this population.

It is my sincere wish that all I have learned on this arduous journey will make the path easier for the many families who will be confronting the autism diagnosis in the future. I hope that in these pages you have found another piece of this mysterious puzzle. The stories in this book are from parents and professionals who are true pioneers dangling on the precipice of violent autism but carrying a dimly lit torch to shine a light upon our lack of knowledge. As we gain clarity, we pass a brighter torch on to you in the hope of illuminating the way for you and the ones you love.

REFERENCES

A child with autism. Retrieved from http://www.child-autism-parent-cafe.com/a-child-with-autism.html

About epilepsy. Retrieved from http://www.epilepsyfoundation.org/aboutepilepsy/index.cfm/types/%20syndromes/infantilespasms.cfm

About Lovaas. ABA for autism. Retrieved from www.lovaascenter.org

Aetna. (n.d.) *Clinical policy bulletin: Pervasive developmental disorders effective: 9.17.2002.* Retrieved from http://www.aetna.com/cpb/medical/data/600_699/0648.html

Amaral, D. G., Schumann, C. M., & Nordahl, C. W. (2008). Neuroanatomy of autism. *Trends Neuroscience, 31*(3), 137-145.

American Psychiatric Association. (2000). *Diagnostic and statistical manual of mental disorders* (4th ed., text rev.). Washington, DC: Author.

Anand, R. (2005). Autism and epilepsy: The complex relationship between cognition, behavior and seizure. *The Internet Journal of Neurology, 4*(1).

Autism history. Retrieved from http://www.news-medical.net/health/Autism-History.aspx

Barr, W. (2003). Is there an epileptic personality? Retrieved from http://www.epilepsy.com/articles/ar_1064250059

Battaglia, A., Parrini, B., & Tancredi, R. (2010, November). The behavioral phenotype of the idic (15) syndrome. *American Journal of Medical Genetics Part C: Seminars in Medical Genetics, 154c*(4), 448-455. Retrieved from http://journals2.scholarportal.info/details.xqy?uri=/15524868/v154ci4/448_tbpotis.xml

Bear, D. M., & Fedio, P. (1977). Quantitative analysis of interictal behavior in temporal lobe epilepsy. *Archives of Neurology, 34*(8), 454-467.

Causes of autism. Retrieved from http://en.wikipedia.org/wiki/Causes_of_autism

The Centers for Disease Control and Prevention. (n.d.). *Autism spectrum disorders, data & statistics.* Retrieved from http://www.cdc.gov/ncbddd/autism/data.html

Characteristics of autism spectrum disorders. Retrieved from http://fiddlefoundation.org

Coben, R., Linden, M., & Myers, T. E (2010). Neurofeedback for autistic spectrum disorder: A review of the literature. *Applied Psychophysiology and Biofeedback, 35*(1), 83-105.

Coben, R., & Padolsky, I. (2007). Assessment-guided neurofeedback for autism spectrum disorder. *Journal of Neurotherapy, 11*(3), 5-18.

Coleman, M., & Blass, J. P. (1985). Autism and lactic acidosis. *Journal of Autism and Developmental Disorders, 15*(1), 1-8. Retrieved from http://www.ncbi.nlm.nih.gov/pubmed/3980425

Cossette, P., Liu, L., Brisebois, K., Dong, H., Lortie, A., Vanasse, M., Saint Hilaire, J. M., Carmant, L., Verner, A., Lu, W. Y., et al. (2011). SYN1-loss-of-function mutations in autism and partial epilepsy cause impaired synaptic function. *Human Molecular Genetics, 20*(12), 2297 2307.

Cowan, J., & Markham, L. (1994, March). *EEG biofeedback for the attention problems of autism: A case study.* Presented at the 25th annual meeting of the Association for Applied Psychophysiology and Biofeedback, Atlanta, GA.

Definition of fetal rubella effects. Retrieved from http://www.medterms.com/script/main/art.asp?articlekey=16130

Depression. Retrieved from http://www.mayoclinic.com/health/depression/DS00175

Deutsch, S. I., Rosse, R. B., Sud, I. M., & Burket, J. A. (2009). Temporal lobe epilepsy confused with panic disorder: Implications for treatment. *Clinical Neuropharmacology, 32*, 160-162.

Edelson, S. (2005). Puberty, aggression and seizures. *Autism Research Review International, 19*(1), 3.

Favors, L. (2009). Electroencephalogram: EEG seizure disorder. Retrieved from http://voices.yahoo.com/electroencephalogram-eeg-seizure-disorder-3771008.html?cat=70

Fetal alcohlol syndrome. Retrieved from http://www.ncbi.nlm.nih.gov/pubmedhealth/PMH0001909/

Fragile X. Retrieved from http://www.fraxa.org

Frombonne, E. (2002). Prevalence of childhood disintegrative disorder. *Autism, 6*(2), 149-157. Retrieved from http://www.asaoakland.org/cdd.htm

Frombonne, E. (2009). Epidemiology of pervasive developmental disorders. *Pediatric Research, 65*(6), 591-598. Retrieved from http://dx.doi.org/10.1203%2FPDR.0b013e31819e7203

Gabis, L., Pomeroy, J., & Andriola, M. R. (2005). Autism and epilepsy: Cause, consequence, comorbidity, or coincidence? *Epilepsy and Behavior, 7*, 652-656.

Gedye, A. (1991). Frontal lobe seizures in autism. *Medical Hypotheses, 34*(2), 174-182.

Genetics overview. Retrieved from www.exploringautism.org

Gibbs, E. L., & Gibbs, F. A. (1951). Electroencephalographic evidence of thalmic or hypothalmic epilepsy. *Neurology, 1*, 138-144.

Gibbs, F. A. (1958). Abnormal electrical activity in the temporal regions and its relationship to abnormalities of behavior. *Research Publications of the Association for Research in Nervous and Mental Disease, 36*, 278-294.

Gillberg, C., & Billstedt, E. (2000). Autism and Asperger syndrome: coexistence with other clinical disorders. *Acta Psychiatrica Scandinavica, 102*, 321-330.

Guerrini, B., Carrozzo, R., Rinaldi, R., & Bonanni, P. (2003). Angelman syndrome: Etiology, clinical features, diagnosis, and management of symptoms. *Paediatric Drugs, 5*(10), 647-661. Retrieved from http://www.ncbi.nlm.nih.gov/pubmed/14510623

Happé F., Ronald A., & Plomin, R. (2006). Time to give up on a single explanation for autism. *Nature Neuroscience, 9*, 1218-1220.

Hara, H. (2007). Autism and epilepsy: A retrospective follow-up study. *Brain Development, 29*, 486-490.

Holmes, G. (2005). Effects of seizures on brain development: Lessons from the laboratory. *Journal of Pediatric Neurology, 33*(1), 1-11. Retrieved from http://www.neurology.org/content/59/9_suppl_5/S3.abstract-content-block#content-block

Hughes, J. R., & John, E. R. (1999). Conventional and quantitative electroencephalography in psychiatry. *Journal of Neuropsychiatry and Clinical Neurosciences, 11*, 190-208.

Hughes, J. R., & Melyn, M. (2005). EEG and seizures in autistic children and adolescents; Further findings with therapeutic implications. *Clinical EEG and Neuroscience, 36*, 15-20.

Hurley, R. A., Fisher, R., & Taber, K. H. (2006). Sudden onset panic: Epileptic aura or panic disorder? *Journal of Neuropsychiatry and Clinical Neurosciences, 18*, 436-443.

Hyperconnectivity. Retrieved from http://en.wikipedia.org

Jarusiewicz, B. (2002). Efficacy of neurofeedback for children in the autistic spectrum: A pilot study. *Journal of Neurotherapy, 6*(4), 39-49.

Johnson, C P., Myers, S. M., & the Council on Children With Disabilities. (2007). Identification and evaluation of children with autism spectrum disorders. *Journal of Pediatrics, 120*(5), 1183-1215. Retrieved from http://aappolicy.aappublications.org/cgi/content/full/pediatrics;120/5/1183#T1

Kanner, L. (1943). Autistic disturbances of affective contact. *Nervous Child, 2*, 217-250.

Kouijzer, M.E.J., de Moor, J.M.H., Gerrits, B.J.L., Buitelaar, J. K., & van Schie, H. T. (2009). Long term effects of neurofeedback treatment in autism. *Research in Autism Spectrum Disorders, 3*(2), 496-501.

Kutscher, M. L. (2006). *Children with seizures: A guide for parents, teachers, and other professionals.* London, UK, and Philadelphia, PA: Jessica Kingsley Publishers.

Landau, W. M., & Keffler, F. R. (1957). Syndrome of acquired aphasia with convulsive disorder in children. *Neurology 7*, 523-530.

LaPlante, E. (1993, 2000). *Seized.* New York, NY: Harper-Collins.

Lennox Gastaut syndrome. Retrieved from http://www.ninds.nih.gov/disorders/lennoxgastautsyndrome/lennoxgastautsyndrome.htm

Libbey, J. E., Sweeten, T. L., McMahon, W. M., & Fujinami, R. S. (2005). Autistic disorder and viral infections. *Journal of Neurovirology, 11*(1), 1-10.

Linden, M., Coben, R., & Myers, T. (2009). Neurofeedback for autism spectrum disorders, A review of the literature. *Applied Psychophysiology and Biofeedback, 35*(1), 83-105.

Lobes of the brain. Retrieved from http://en.wikipedia.org/wiki/File:Lobes_of_the_brain.jpg

Marikar, S., Childs, D., & Chitale, R. (2009). Death certificate: John Travolta's teen son died of a seizure. Retrieved from http://abcnews.go.com/Entertainment/MindMoodNews/story?id=6584462&page=1

Martell, A. (2006). *Getting Adam back.* Retrieved from http://epilepsymoms.com/book-review-of-getting-adam-back

Miranda, F. (n.d.). Retrieved from http://www.brightmindsinstitute.com

Munoz-Yunta, J. A., Salvado, B., Ortiz-Alonso, T., Amo, C., Fernandez-Lucas, A., Maestu, F., & Palau-Baduell, M. (2003, February). Clinical features of epilepsy in autism spectrum disorders. *Review of Neurology*, 36 Suppl 1:S61-7. Retrieved from http://www.ncbi.nlm.nih.gov/pubmed/12599105

National Dissemination Center for Children With Disabilities (NICHCY). (2011). *IDEA: The Individuals with Disabilities Education Act*. Retrieved from http://nichcy.org/laws/idea

Neurofeedback guidelines for parents. Retrieved from www.jacobsassociates.org

Neurofeedback helps those with autistic disorders, study finds (Feb. 26, 2008). *Science Daily*. Retrieved from http://www.sciencedaily.com/releases/2008/02/080226185848.htm

Newschaffer, C. J., Croen, L. A., Daniels, J., et al. (2007). The epidemiology of autism spectrum disorders. *Annual Review of Public Health, 28*, 235-258. Retrieved from http://dx.doi.org/10.1146%2Fannurev.publhealth.28.021406.144007

Nyhan, W. L. (2005, September-October). Disorders of purine and pyrimidine metabolism. *Molecular Genetics and Metabolism, 86*(1-2), 25-33. Retrieved from http://www.ncbi.nlm.nih.gov/pubmed/16176880

Philpot, B., Mabb, A., & Judson, M. (2011). *Insights for autism from Angelman syndrome*. Retrieved from http://sfari.org/news-and-opinion/viewpoint/2011/insights-for-autism-from-angelman-syndromee

Progressive myoclonic epilepsies. Retrieved from http://www.epilepsy.com/epilepsy/epilepsy_promyoclonic

Refrigerator mothers. (2006). Retrieved from http://autism.about. com/od/causesofautism/p/refrigerator.htm

Restak, R. (1995). Complex partial seizures present diagnostic challenge. *Psychiatric Times, 12,* 9. Retrieved from www.psychiatrictimes.com/display/article/10168/54456

Rett syndrome. Retrieved from http://en.wikipedia.org/wiki/Rett_syndrome

Reynolds, T., & Dombeck, M. (2006). *Historical/contemporary theories of cause and genetic contributions.* Retrieved from www.mentalhelp.net/poc/view_doc.php?type=doc&id=8771&cn=20

Rimland, B., & Edelson, S. M. (2000). *Autism treatment evaluation checklist (ATEC).* Retrieved from http://autismeval.com/ari-atec/report1.html

Rubenstein-Taybi syndrome; caused by mutations in the transcriptional co-activator CBP. Retrieved from http://www.ncbi. nlm.nih.gov/pubmed/7630403

Seizures, what everyone with a child on the spectrum should know. (2010). Retrieved from http://www.tacanow.org/family-resources/seizures/

Shipman, C., & Nalty, A. (2008). The answers to autism may be inside the mind. Retrieved from http://abcnews.go.com/GMA/OnCall/story?id=4882297 &page=2

Smith-Magenis syndrome. Retrieved from http://www.ncbi.nlm. nih.gov/books/NBK1310/

Tammet, D. (2007). *Born on a blue day.* New York, NY: Free Press.

References

Thompson, L., Thompson, M., & Reid, A. (2010). Neurofeedback outcomes in clients with Asperger's syndrome. *Applied Psychophysiological Biofeedback, 35*(1), 63-81.

Thompson, S. A., Duncan, J. S., & Shelagh, S. M. (2000). Partial seizures presenting as panic attacks. *British Medical Journal, 321,* 1002-1003.

Treffert, D. A. (1964). The psychiatric patient with an EEG temporal lobe focus. *The American Journal of Psychiatry, 120,* 765-771.

Treffert, D. A. (2009). The savant syndrome: An extraordinary condition. A synopsis: past, present, future. *Philosophical Transactions of the Royal Society B Biological Sciences, 364*(1522), 1351-1357. Retrieved from http://rstb.royalsocietypublishing.org/content/364/1522/1351.full

Tropea, D., Giacometti, E., Wilson, N., Beard C., et al. (2009). Partial reversal of Rett syndrome-like symptoms in MeCP2 mutant mice. *Proceedings of the National Academy of Science, 106,* 2029-2034.

Tuchman, R., Alessandri, M., & Cuccaro, M. (2010). Autism and epilepsy: Historical perspective. *Brain and Development, 32,* 709-718.

Types of seizures. Retrieved from http://www.fiddlefoundation.org

Volkmar, R. M., & Rutter, M. (1995). Childhood disintegrative disorder: Results of the DSM-1V autism field trial. *Journal of the American Academy of Child and Adolescent Psychiatry, 34,* 1092-1095.

Waxman, S. G., & Geschwind, N. (1975). The interictal behavior syndrome in temporal lobe epilepsy. *Archives of General Psychiatry, 32*(12), 1580-1586.

Wazana, A., Bresnahan, M., & Kline, J. (2007). The autism epidemic: Fact or artifact? *Journal of the American Academy of Child & Adolescent Psychiatry, 46*(6), 721-730.

What is autism? Retrieved from http://www.acesautism.com/faq.html

Williams, D. (1998). *Nobody nowhere*. Philadelphia, PA: Jessica Kingsley Publishers.

Williams, D. (2010). My experiences with atypical epilepsy. An interview/blog. Retrieved from http://blog.donnawilliams.net

Wing, L., & Potter D. (2002). The epidemiology of autistic spectrum disorders: Is the true prevalence rising? *Mental Retardation and Developmental Disabilities Research Review, 8*(3), 151-161.

Young, G. B., Chandarana, M. B., Blume, W. T., McLachlan, R. S., Munoz, D. G., & Girvin, J. P. (1995). Mesial temporal seizures presenting as anxiety disorders. *Journal of Neuropsychiatry, 7*, 352-357.

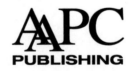

PUBLISHING

P.O. Box 23173
Shawnee Mission, Kansas 66283-0173
www.aapcpublishing.net